Colour Atlas of
Mesothelioma

Commission of the European Communities

Colour Atlas of Mesothelioma

Prepared for the Commission of the European Communities, Directorate-General Employment, Social Affairs and Education, Industrial Medicine and Hygiene Division, by

J.S.P. Jones

Department of Pathology,
City Hospital,
Nottingham, United Kingdom

C. Lund

Patologisk Institut,
Centralsygehuset,
Holstebro, Denmark

H.T. Planteydt

Streeklaboratorium 'Zeeland',
Middelburg, The Netherlands

with a section on Cytology of Effusions by
E.B. Butler

Department of Pathology,
St Mary's Hospital,
Manchester, United Kingdom

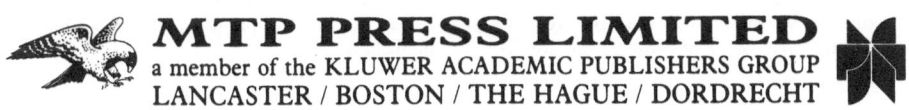

MTP PRESS LIMITED
a member of the KLUWER ACADEMIC PUBLISHERS GROUP
LANCASTER / BOSTON / THE HAGUE / DORDRECHT

Published in the UK and Europe by
MTP Press Limited
Falcon House
Lancaster, England

British Library Cataloguing in Publication Data

Jones, J.S.P.
  Colour atlas of mesothelioma.
  1. Mesothelioma
  I. Title II. Lund, C. III. Planteydt, H.T.
  IV. Series
  616.99'4   RC280.L8

  ISBN-13: 978-94-011-7317-9

Published in the USA by
MTP Press
A division of Kluwer Boston Inc
190 Old Derby Street
Hingham, MA 02043, USA

Library of Congress Cataloging in Publication Data

Jones, J.S.P., 1929–
  Colour atlas of mesothelioma.

  Bibliography: p.
  Includes index.
  1. Mesothelioma—Atlases. 2. Histology, Pathological
—Atlases. I. Lund, C., 1938–   II. Planteydt,
H.T., 1927–   III. Commission of the European
Communities. Industrial Medicine and Hygiene Division.
IV. Title. [DNLM: 1. Mesothelioma—atlases. QZ 17 C7196]
RC280.L8J66 1984   616.99'2   84–21281
ISBN-13: 978-94-011-7317-9   e-ISBN-13: 978-94-011-7315-5
DOI: 10.1007/978-94-011-7315-5

Publication arranged by
Commission of the European Communities,
Directorate-General Information Market and Innovation,
Luxembourg

EUR 9216 EN

Trowbridge, Wiltshire

Contents

Foreword

by W.J. Hunter

In 1977 a report of a Working Group of experts prepared for the Commission of the European Communities was published entitled 'Public Health Risks of Exposure to Asbestos' (EUR 5653e)[1]. This report contained several conclusions and recommendations; one of the latter stated that 'a mesothelioma register should be set up in those countries of the EEC where none exist, in accordance with criteria and procedures agreed upon by a panel of pathologists'.

Acting upon this recommendation, the Commission established a C.E.C. Mesothelioma Panel, which has as one of its basic objectives the standardization of the pathological diagnosis of mesotheliomas, by exchange of information between members of National Panels.

Since its establishment, several meetings have been held, and much useful information has been exchanged. This work has been underlined by the adoption by the Council of Ministers of a Directive on the protection of workers from the risks related to asbestos at work[2] which requires Member States to keep a register of recognized cases of mesothelioma.

To assist Member States in the establishment of such registers, the Commission of the European Communities considered it would be useful for an illustrated book on mesotheliomas to be prepared. Three pathologists who are members of the C.E.C. Mesothelioma Panel have undertaken this task and this publication is the result. The material used has mostly been derived from cases submitted to the C.E.C. Panel, but some contributions have come from other sources.

It is hoped that this publication will help all who are involved in keeping a Register of Mesotheliomas, and it is also hoped that those who have an interest in this area will find this mesothelioma atlas of value.

[1] 'Zielhuis Report'. Pergamon Press, Oxford.
[2] O.J. of the European Communities L 263 of 24 Sept. 1983, pp. 25–32.

Introduction

This *Colour Atlas of Mesothelioma* has been written and illustrated by pathologists for their fellow pathologists in the hope that this information will be of help in making the pathological diagnosis of diffuse malignant mesothelioma. Short sections on clinical aspects, aetiology and epidemiology have been added. Apart from the systematic text and illustrations, case reports have been used to highlight some of the problems in diagnosis.

As many countries now have Mesothelioma Panels, information on these Panels and on their aims has been included. The addresses are as complete as possible and represent the situation in the year 1984.

The sections on pathogenesis and on diagnostic developments have been kept deliberately short because these subjects will be especially liable to review in future years.

The term mesothelioma is used in the literature for tumours other than diffuse malignant mesothelioma. A chapter has been included in order to emphasize that these tumours are separate entities.

Certain references are given at the end of the relevant sections and a more comprehensive list may be obtained from the bibliography.

We would like to thank all our colleagues who have supplied us with valuable material. Without their help we could not have prepared this Atlas.

J.S.P. Jones
C. Lund
H.T. Planteydt

Acknowledgements

We would like to thank all the members of our technical and secretarial staff for their help in the preparation of this Atlas. We are particularly indebted to Mr W. Brackenbury for his skilful microphotography and to Mr G.B. Gilbert for preparing the illustrations. We would especially like to thank Mrs V.G. Bolton for preparing the many drafts and the final manuscript of the Atlas.

August 1984   J.S.P. Jones
                                                     C. Lund
                                                     H.T. Planteydt

1

Mesothelioma: Definition and Considerations

A mesothelioma is a neoplasm of the mesothelium. The mesothelium is the cellular lining of the original coelomic cavities, including their derivates and remnants. From a practical point of view, it is the mesotheliomas of the greater serosal cavities that are of major importance, the rest being of lesser interest, but they all take a natural place within the limits of this atlas. For this reason the atlas is mainly devoted to DIFFUSE MALIGNANT MESOTHELIOMA of the PLEURA, PERITONEUM and PERICARDIUM. Other forms of 'mesothelioma' are dealt with briefly at the end of the atlas.

Since the total group of mesotheliomas is very heterogenic, the definitions and biological behaviour of the subgroups are considered separately under their different headings.

2

The Mesothelium

I. EMBRYOLOGY

In the early somite stage of the developing embryo, multiple coelomic spaces are formed (Figure 1). Each of these spaces is enclosed by mesoblasts which are derived from the intra-embryonic mesoderm. The mesoblasts differentiate into a single layer of mesothelium. The cavities fuse to form a single continuous coelomic cavity. As a result of invagination of organs and various fusions, the single cavity becomes separated into the pericardial, pleural and peritoneal cavities, and also the tunica vaginalis. The differentiation of mesoblasts takes place at a later stage than other mesodermal developments, such as differentiation into vascular endothelium, muscles etc.

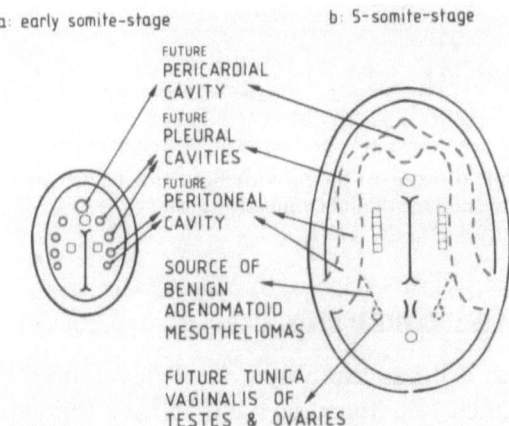

Figure 1 Embryonic disc, dorsal view, showing development of coelomic cavities (shaded)

3

II. HISTOLOGY, CYTOLOGY AND ULTRASTRUCTURE

The mesothelium is a cellular monolayer composed of flattened, interlocking, polygonal cells (squames), (Figure 2), joined together by zonulae occludentes and/or desmosomes. The cytoplasm may in places be as little as 0.1 μm thick, and the nucleus usually bulges into the overlying space. The cells bear scattered microvilli and one or two cilia on their free surfaces. Micropinocytic vesicles are common in the cytoplasm, which is otherwise relatively poorly provided with organelles. Several structural variants of the mesothelial cells have been recognized – one type probably being the stem cell.

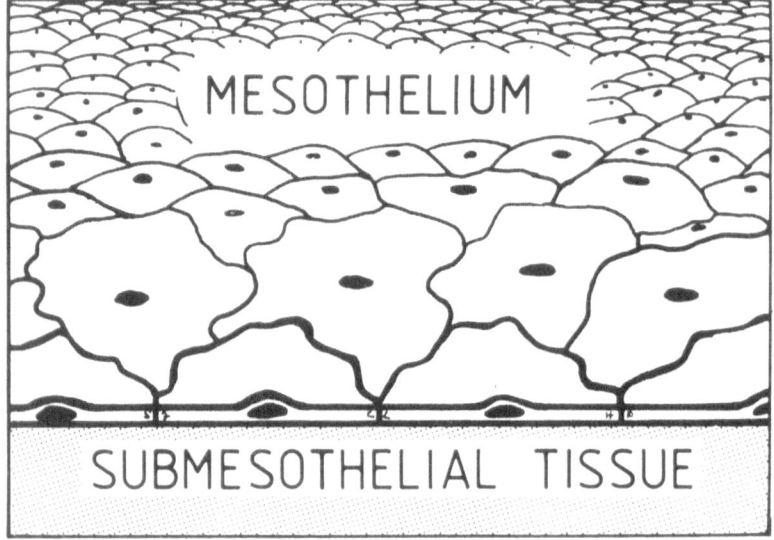

Figure 2   Schematic drawing of the mesothelium as a pavement squamous monolayer resting on the submesothelial connective tissue

III. CELLULAR PROPERTIES

The mesothelial cell has the potential of developing along at least two separate lines. On the one hand it may follow an epithelial pathway, while on the other a connective tissue development may be pursued. This is demonstrated in tissue cultures, in inflammation and in neoplasia. It has also been claimed that the mesothelial cell possesses a phagocytic capability, and may leave the surface to form a free macrophage.

IV. SUBMESOTHELIAL TISSUE

The mesothelium rests upon a 30–40 nm thick basal lamina, under which there is connective tissue with a varying amount of elastic fibrils. For the visceral pleura this connective tissue rests on the elastic lamina covering the lung, while in the parietal pleura, peritoneum and pericardium, it is directly continuous with the neighbouring soft tissues.

References

Behbehani, A.M., Hunter, W.J., Chapman, A.L. and Lin, F. (1982). Studies of a human mesothelioma. *Hum. Pathol.* **13**, 862–866

Ham, A.W. and Cormark, D.H. (1979). *Histology*. Edn. 8, Ch. 8. (Philadelphia: Lippincott)

Spencer, H. (1977). *Pathology of the Lung*. 3rd Edn. pp. 6 and 69 (Oxford: Pergamon)

Williams, P.L. and Warwick, R. (Eds.). (1980). *Gray's Anatomy*. 36th Edn. Chapter 2. (Edinburgh: Churchill Livingstone)

3

Diffuse Malignant Mesothelioma (of pleura, peritoneum and pericardium)

I. GROSS PATHOLOGY

Mesothelioma is classically a diffuse tumour which has a dense white appearance, but occasionally it has a yellow or grey coloration. The consistency is variable, but usually the tumour is hard. Necrosis is not a common finding. The growth pattern is typically sheet-like but sometimes it is also nodular and even papillary. It is not uncommon for the tumour to be multifocal. The thickness may vary from a few millimetres to several centimetres.

It grows along the serosal membranes of the pleura, peritoneum or pericardium and in its early stages it is seen as a thin sheet which may involve either the visceral or parietal layers of the body cavities. Usually a straw-coloured effusion is present in the initial stages, but as the tumour grows, the space between the two layers of the serosal surfaces becomes progressively obliterated. There may be loculation of fluid before the cavities become completely overtaken by neoplasm. Occasionally fluid may persist throughout the course of the disease; in other instances fluid formation does not occur at any stage.

(a) Pleura

This is the commonest site for diffuse malignant mesotheliomas. The tumour becomes firmly fixed on to the lining wall of the chest and it is locked into the intercostal muscles, often compressing the inter-costal nerves. The tumour also becomes firmly adherent to the surface of the lung leaving no plane of cleavage. This makes a meso-thelioma very difficult to remove and this is a characteristic feature at surgery and at autopsy. The mesothelioma may occupy the entire pleural surface, totally encasing the lung in an envelope of rigid tumour. It also classically grows along the interlobar serosal surfaces, forming a thin white sheet of tumour.

(b) Peritoneum

Mesothelioma may present as a primary tumour of the peritoneum. It forms sheets of dense white tissue which in the beginning selective-ly appear along the serosal surfaces of the viscera. These gradually merge with each other, and later the tumour on the visceral and parietal layers of the peritoneum becomes completely confluent, ending with a 'frozen' peritoneal cavity. Characteristically the serosal tumour does not invade through the muscle and mucosal layers of the gastro-intestinal tract and even in the most advanced cases there is no disturbance to the normal pattern of mucosal folds in the stomach and intestines.

The individual organs within the abdominal cavity may become completely encased in tumour, but there is characteristically only limited infiltration into the underlying tissues.

In early peritoneal mesothelioma there may be a single source of tumour, or there may be multiple separate tumours which later merge to form the more diffuse pattern described above. Large amounts of ascitic fluid may be produced, especially in the early stages, but the quantity of fluid often diminishes as the tumour increasingly occupies the intra-abdominal space.

(c) Pericardium

Primary pericardial mesothelioma is exceptionally rare. It can only be diagnosed if there is no primary tumour in any other site, includ-ing the pleura and peritoneum. The tumour may involve the visceral pericardium in thick bands encapsulating the heart and showing invasion of the underlying myocardium. The parietal pericardium may also be involved, in which case there may be nodular projections into the pericardial cavity. A haemorrhagic pericardial effusion is a common feature, but if both layers of pericardium are involved they may fuse and obliterate the cavity.

(d) Metastases

(i) Direct

Although the growth of the mesothelioma is essentially one of diffuse involvement of the primary serosal surface, the depth of invasion into neighbouring structures is relatively limited. However because of the large area of serosal surfaces that are involved in the primary growth, it is inevitable that large areas of the body are subjected to direct invasion, however shallow this may be. For example in pleural mesothelioma the inner lining of the entire chest wall may show invasion; in peritoneal mesothelioma the outer muscle layer of the entire alimentary tract may be affected.

Direct spread of the tumour may occur through the diaphragm. Spread may also occur to the pericardium and to the opposite pleural cavity. If a surgical procedure has been carried out, the mesothelioma may spread along the incision to form a subcutaneous tumour mass.

(ii) Transcoelomic

It is not certain whether mesothelioma arises as a multifocal neoplastic process which is followed by the merging together of the multiple islands of tumour on the serosal surface, or whether there is a single primary source followed by multifocal implantation of seedling deposits derived from the tumour cells which are floating in the effusions. It is probable that both mechanisms occur. In many cases, more than one serosal cavity is involved.

(iii) Lymphatic

Mesothelioma frequently invades lymph vessels and spreads to regional lymph nodes. Within the chest cavity it is relatively common to see macroscopic evidence of tumour spread within the peribronchial lymph vessels, so that a cuff of white tumour tissue forms a rigid tube around the bronchi.

Pulmonary and mediastinal lymph nodes are often invaded. Para-aortic lymph nodes may be invaded from both peritoneal and pleural primary mesotheliomas.

(iv) Blood-borne

Mesothelioma generally shows little tendency to blood-borne metastases. They do occur however in lung, liver, bone, kidney, adrenal gland, brain, muscle, myocardium, skin etc.

(e) Differential diagnosis

In making the diagnosis of mesothelioma, the gross findings are of paramount importance, but a definite diagnosis can only be made on histological examination.

It is necessary to differentiate between diffuse malignant mesothelioma and

(i) reactive processes affecting serosal membranes,
(ii) malignant tumours other than mesothelioma.

(i) Reactive processes affecting serosal membranes

Fibrosis, causing considerable thickening of the pleura, can mimic a mesothelioma. However it usually has a shiny appearance on examination of the cut surface due to hyalinization. Another common feature is the sharp demarcation between lung and pleura. These features are less distinct if an active inflammation is present. In severe cases of pleural fibrosis the lung may be totally encased.

Pleural plaques are yellow-white patchy thickened areas of the parietal pleura, which project slightly above the surrounding tissue and have a shiny porcelain-like appearance. They may be flat or nodular, but they all have a smooth surface. A wide variety of shapes and sizes is seen. The consistency is like articular cartilage, but it may be brittle if the plaques are calcified.

Plaques are classically situated on the posterior wall of the lower chest, usually along the lines of the ribs and also on the central tendon of the diaphragm. They may also be present in the paravertebral region.

(ii) Malignant tumours other than mesothelioma

The exclusion of a primary carcinoma of any organ by a carefully conducted examination is an important factor in making a positive diagnosis of mesothelioma. The reluctance to show deep infiltration either into lung tissue or into stomach or bowel wall, provides further supportive evidence that the neoplasm is a mesothelioma rather than a secondary carcinoma. Primary or secondary connective tissue tumours can mimic a mesothelioma but they tend to form a more circumscribed and nodular type of infiltrative neoplasm rather than spreading relatively thinly along serosal membranes. Likewise, lymphomatous tumours are more rounded and they form softer, white, fleshy masses. The distribution of the lymphoma in the mediastinum or in the posterior abdominal region, rather than on the serosal surface gives an additional aid to differential diagnosis.

II. HISTOPATHOLOGY

(a) Growth pattern

The most characteristic feature of this tumour – its diffuse growth along the serosal surface – is seen at microscopic level as well as in the gross specimen.

In rare instances very small mesotheliomas can occur on a macroscopically normal serosa. Initially abnormal cells replace the mesothelium. At a later stage when the tumours are larger, there is growth both above and below the original mesothelial level. In the visceral pleura the subpleural elastic layer remains intact even after considerable extension of the tumour. Ultimately, neoplasm may invade . the elastic layer, so involving the underlying lung parenchyma. In the case of the parietal layer of the pleura, and in both parietal and visceral layers of the peritoneum and pericardium, there is shallow, uniform invasion of the adjacent connective tissue.

Sometimes inclusion of the pre-existing lung tissue is found in the tumour. This explains the presence of alveolar macrophages and asbestos bodies in the tumour.

The tumour may be found in relation to pleural plaques, either next to the plaque, or covering it on the serosal side, growing underneath it, or sometimes actually infiltrating the plaque.

In advanced cases the tumour invades the lymphatic system, and on rare occasions blood vessels.

(b) Histological features

The characteristic feature in the histopathology of mesothelioma is the wide variation in the pattern of the tumour and the presence of epithelial and connective tissue differentiation. This provides the basis for description of the following types according to the dominating features.

(i) Epithelial type,
(ii) Connective tissue type,
(iii) Mixed type.

(i) Epithelial type

This shows tubular, papillary and tubulo-papillary structures of a wide variety of patterns, including clefts, solid nests and sheets. Loose groups of epithelial cells can be found and also undifferentiated areas. In some cases an abundant, oedematous, mucoid stroma is found with relatively small numbers of loosely arranged tumour cells with poorly formed tubules, clefts and cystic spaces. The papillary structures may have connective tissue stalks, while the tubules and clefts are usually surrounded by dense collagen bundles. Amyloid deposits have been described. Squamous metaplasia of the epithelial type tumour has been found on rare occasions.

The cellular features show regularity in most cases, in contrast to the variability of histological architecture. The epithelial type cells are cuboidal or polyhedral, occasionally flat or low cylindrical. Two types of epithelial cells can be distinguished.

(1) Small cells with a moderate amount of acidophilic cytoplasm. The small nuclei are oval or round with a rather heavy nuclear membrane with pale, uniformly distributed chromatin and small nucleoli.

(2) Larger cells with weakly acidophilic or basophilic cytoplasm. The nuclei are moderately large and vesicular and they have prominent nucleoli.

Usually one cell type is found, but mixtures and intermediate forms occur. Occasionally binucleation, and even multinucleation is present. The number of mitoses is low. Pleomorphism, anaplasia and atypical mitoses are rare. Areas of closely packed spheroidal or polygonal cells may occur, sometimes with plentiful acidophilic or amphophilic cytoplasm. Extensive sheets of these cells may occur without tubulo-papillary structures. Nuclei may be eccentric. Rarely, some tumours contain psammoma bodies in the epithelial parts. Similar but more irregular calcified structures also may occur. In many epithelial type tumours, vacuoles or cystic spaces occur. Special stains are necessary to investigate these latter structures.

(ii) Connective tissue type

This consists of bundles of fibroblast-like cells alternating with areas in which very few nuclei are found. Small foci of atypical cells are also present. The proportion of cells to collagen varies and often large areas are found which are mainly collagenous and may even be completely hyalinized. The collagen often has a characteristic pattern with irregularly orientated spindle-shaped clefts, sometimes lined by tumour cells. Fine strands of hyaline collagen form complex mesh works, not found in other tumours or fibrous reactions. On the other hand some areas may be very cellular. Vacuoles or cystic spaces rarely occur. The non-collagenous intercellular substance varies in amount and staining properties.

The cells of the connective tissue type of mesothelioma are oval, somewhat elongated, fusiform or spindle shaped. The oval cells resemble the epithelial type cells and have the same vesicular nuclei. Sometimes it is difficult to determine whether solid nests are groups of epithelial type tumour cells or bundles of spindle cells cut perpendicularly to the longitudinal axis. Anaplasia and pleomorphism may also be present in a connective tissue type mesothelioma. The connective tissue type occasionally shows special differentiation into fibrosarcomatous, myosarcomatous, chondrosarcomatous, or osteosarcomatous forms.

The connective tissue type of mesothelioma is often referred to in the literature as the sarcomatous, sarcomatoid, spindle cell, mesenchymal, desmoplastic or fibrous type.

(iii) Mixed type

This shows features of both epithelial and connective tissue types, and indeed the majority of mesotheliomas have this dimorphic histological appearance. The two components may be present together or there may be a dominance of one type in one part of the tumour with the other component predominating in another area.

A common feature of all three types is the rarity with which necrosis is found. Aggregates of lymphocytes may be present in variable amounts in all three types.

(iv) Metastases

The histological and cellular features of the metastases of diffuse malignant mesothelioma show the same variation as can be found in the primary tumours. In the majority of cases the type of the metastasis is similar to that in the primary tumour. However the predominant differentiation in the metastases can be different from that in the primary tumour, e.g. a mainly connective tissue type of mesothelioma can show in its metastases a mainly epithelial differentiation, and vice versa.

(c) Special stains

The following stains are recommended in the diagnosis and differential diagnosis of diffuse malignant mesothelioma.

(1) Periodic Acid Schiff stain (PAS).
(2) Periodic Acid Schiff stain after diastase pre-treatment (diastase–PAS).
(3) Reticulin stain (e.g. Gomori's reticulin stain).
(4) Van Gieson stain for collagen.
(5) Alcian Blue with and without hyaluronidase. This is recommended with some reservation as it is extremely important to

do the stain at the correct pH of 2.5; also different kinds of hyaluronidase may give different results.

In the interpretation of the PAS stain the role of the fixative should be considered. False negative results are obtained if water-soluble substances are removed by the process of fixation. In many mesotheliomas small PAS-positive granules are found which are removed by pre-treatment with diastase. This glycogen can be found in epithelial as well as in connective tissue type tumours. Sometimes, after pre-treatment with diastase, weakly positive granules are found in the cytoplasm of the epithelial type tumour cells. Connective tissue elements in the tumour may also be found weakly positive using the diastase–PAS stain. The presence of mucin, especially in the form of diastase–PAS-positive globules in the cytoplasm of tumour cells, excludes a mesothelioma. The large vacuoles in the cytoplasm of the epithelial type of mesothelioma all appear empty, not only in the H & E stained sections, but also in those stained with PAS. However they may contain alcian blue-positive material, but this disappears after pre-treatment with hyaluronidase. The presence of this hyaluronic acid is considered diagnostic only when found in epithelial type tumour cells. Stromal hyaluronic acid is more prominent in mesotheliomas than in other conditions but this feature is not exclusively diagnostic.

In sheets of epithelial type tumour cells, scanty reticulin fibres are found which surround groups of cells or individual cells. A more intimate framework of reticulin fibres is found in a mesothelioma than in a carcinoma.

The Van Gieson stain is used to estimate the amount of hyaline collagen. If myomatous differentiation is suspected a supplementary PTAH stain is recommended, although this stain rarely reveals characteristic features by light microscopy.

(d) Diagnostic histopathological criteria

The diagnosis of diffuse malignant mesothelioma is preferably based upon the presence of both epithelial and connective tissue types of structures, or on the presence of other combinations, e.g. various differentiations of connective tissue type or combinations with undifferentiated tumour areas. Several of these combinations are considered diagnostic or at least highly suggestive. Evidence of mesothelial differentiation is always considered diagnostic. When the amount of tissue available for examination is small, the chances of seeing the variation of tumour patterns will be limited, e.g. one may see only connective tissue type tumour or only epithelial elements. Both can be derived from a mixed type of mesothelioma. If these are both found in one biopsy specimen the diagnosis is certain. Adequate sampling or multiple biopsies are therefore very important. Pleural, peritoneal and pericardial diffuse malignant mesotheliomas show the same spectrum of variation in the histopathological specimens, although some preference of the epithelial type of peritoneal tumours has been reported.

(e) Differential diagnosis

In histopathology as well as in gross pathology it is necessary to differentiate between diffuse malignant mesothelioma and

(i) reactive processes affecting serosal membranes,
(ii) malignant tumours other than mesothelioma.

(i) Reactive processes affecting serosal membranes

Fibrosis without specific features is usually poor in cells but it may contain some lymphocytes. The border with the adjacent tissues may be irregular, but usually there is a sharp demarcation between lung parenchyma and pleural fibrosis. Hyalinization and calcified areas are common features. Residual islands of mesothelial proliferation of epithelial type may occur in the fibrous tissue, but these are limited to the level of the pre-existing serosal membrane. In these cases the differential diagnosis between reaction and tumour may be very difficult. Acute cellular-rich, 'productive' pleuritis may be an important differential diagnosis, but here the presence of granulation tissue is a diagnostic feature together with 'layering' of the fibrotic organization.

Reactive mesothelial cell proliferation may occur under different conditions such as inflammation, circulatory disturbances, lung infarction, and cirrhosis of the liver. Papillary formations of hyperplastic epithelial-like mesothelium may then cover the serosal surfaces, even over large areas. Usually the cells have regular nuclei and cytoplasm, but they can be atypical.

Pleural plaques consist of parallel-running hyaline collagen fibres, poor in nuclei, and with a 'basket weave' and avascular appearance. Calcification may occur. The plaques can be found in the neighbourhood of mesotheliomas or they may be surrounded or invaded by mesothelioma. In the connective tissue type of mesothelioma, the collagen fibres may be arranged in bundles, but they are not as consistently parallel as those seen in pleural plaques.

(ii) Malignant tumours other than mesothelioma

The epithelial type of mesothelioma and the epithelial component of a mixed type can be difficult to distinguish from metastatic adenocarcinoma.

In differentiating mesothelioma from peripheral lung carcinoma, an intact elastic layer is found in many cases of mesothelioma, but not in peripheral lung carcinoma invading the pleura. Usually metastases are more multi-nodular than mesothelioma, and the presence of epithelial mucin, demonstrated by the diastase–PAS stain, excludes a mesothelioma. Psammoma bodies may occur in mesothelioma but are much more frequent in metastases of carcinoma especially from the ovary, lung and thyroid. Secondary carcinoma in the pleura or in the peritoneum from a primary tumour of one of these three organs may be very difficult to distinguish from a mesothelioma, grossly as well as microscopically. Glycogen is usually present in cytoplasm of the tumour cells in metastases from carcinomas of the kidney and testis, as well as in mesotheliomas.

Although the presence of a mixed pattern is decisive for the diagnosis of mesothelioma there remains a small group of cases in which no definite conclusion can be drawn even after considering the histopathology in combination with the clinical data and a thorough macroscopic examination.

The connective tissue type of mesothelioma may be difficult to differentiate from a sarcoma, in particular a fibrosarcoma, leiomyosarcoma or a vascular tumour. When metastases from kidney carcinomas show sarcomatous areas with spindle cells, the differentiation may be very difficult.

The mixed type of mesothelioma. The only differential diagnostic problem may lie in the very rare possibility of a metastasis from a synovial sarcoma.

References

Abelanet, R., Hagueus, M., Fondimare, A. and Roujeau, J. (1979). Les méso-théliomes pleuraux. *Rev.Fr.Mal.Resp.,* **7**, 243–264

Andersen, J.A. and Hansen, B.F. (1974). Primary pericardial mesothelioma. *Dan.Med.Bull.,* **21**, No. 5, 195–200

Andrion, A., Colombo, A., Dacorsi, M. and Mollo, F. (1982). Pleural plaques at autopsy in Turin – a study of 1019 adult subjects. *Eur.J.Respir.Dis.,* **63**, 107–112

Antman, K.H. (1980). Current concepts – malignant mesothelioma. *N.Engl. J.Med.,* **303**, 200–202 and 1303–1304

Berge, T. and Lundberg, S. (1977). Cancer in Malmö 1958–1969. An autopsy study. *Acta Path. Microbiol.Scand.,* Section A, Suppl.260

Cantin, R., Al-Jabi, M. and McCaughey, W.T.E. (1982). Desmoplastic diffuse mesothelioma. *Am.J.Surg.Pathol.,* **6**, 215–222

Edstrom, L.E., Dawson, P.J., Kohler, J. and de Meester, T.R. (1980). Malignant mesothelioma: a metastasis to the face. *J.Surg.Oncol.,* **14**, 251–254

Fisher, E.R. and Hellstrom, H.R. (1960). The periodic acid–schiff reaction as an aid in the identification of mesothelioma. *Cancer,* **13**, No. 4, 837–841

Gellert, A.R. and Steel, S.J. (1982). Pleural mesothelioma: diagnosis by trephine biopsy. *Br.J.Dis.Chest.,* **76**, 303

Goldstein, B. (1979). Two malignant pleural mesotheliomas with unusual histological features. *Thorax,* **34**, 375–379

Griffiths, M.H., Riddell, R.J. and Xipell, J.M., (1980). Malignant mesothelioma; a review of 35 cases with diagnosis and prognosis. *Pathology,* **12**, 591–603

Herbert, A. and Gallagher, P.J. (1982). Pleural biopsy in the diagnosis of malignant mesothelioma. *Thorax,* **37**, 816–821

Hillerdal, G. (1983). Pleural plaques in Sweden among immigrants from Finland – with an editorial note. *Eur.J.Resp.Dis.,* **64**, 391–392

Hillerdal, G. and Lindgren, A. (1980). Pleural plaques: correlation of autopsy findings to radiographic findings and occupational history. *Eur.J.Respir.Dis.,* **61**, 315–319

Hourihane, D.O'B. (1964). The pathology of mesotheliomata and an analysis of their association with asbestos exposure. *Thorax,* **19**, 268–278

Kannerstein, M., Churg, J. and Magner, D. (1973). Histochemistry in the diagnosis of mesothelioma. *Ann.Clin.Lab.Sci.,* **3**, 207–211

Kannerstein, M. and Churg, J. (1977). Peritoneal mesothelioma. *Hum.Pathol.,* **8**, 83–94

Lajartre, A.Y., Mussini-Montpellier, J. and Lenne, Y. (1976). Étude anatomo-pathologique de 54 cas de mésothéliomes pleuraux diffus observés dans les régions portuaires de Nantes, Saint Nazaire et Lorient. *Ann. Anat.Pathol.Paris,* **21**, No. 2, 247–260

Law, M.R., Hodson, M.E. and Heard, B.E. (1982). Malignant mesothelioma of the pleura: relation between histological type and clinical behaviour. *Thorax,* **37**, 810–815

McCaughey, W.T.E. (1965). Criteria for diagnosis of diffuse mesothelial tumours. *Ann.N.Y.Acad.Sci.,* **132**, 603–613

Mahaim, I. (1945). *Les Tumeurs et les Polypes du Coeur.* (Paris: Masson et Cie)

Sills, M., Segal, E. and Spitzer, S.A. (1983). Trephine drill biopsy in the diagnosis of malignant pleural mesothelioma. *Eur.J.Resp.Dis.,* **64,** 391–392

Sytman, A.L. and Mac-Alpin, R.N. (1971). Primary pericardial mesothelioma. Report of three cases and review of the literature. *Am.Heart J.,* **81,** 760–769

Wagner, J.C., Munday, D.E. and Harington, J.S. (1962). Histochemical demonstration of hyaluronic acid in pleural mesotheliomas. *J.Pathol.Bact.,* **84,** No. 1, 73–78

Whitwell, F. and Rawcliffe, R.M. (1971). Diffuse malignant pleural mesothelioma and asbestos exposure. *Thorax,* **26,** 6–22

Yilling, F.P., Schlant, R.C., Hertzler, G.L. and Krzyaniak, R. (1982). Pericardial mesothelioma. *Chest,* **81,** (4), 520–523

III. CYTOLOGY OF EFFUSIONS, ASPIRATES AND IMPRINTS

Cytology of effusions

The extent to which cells exfoliate into effusions depends on the stage of the disease and on the type of mesothelioma. In the early stages histiocytes and lymphocytes are common, without exfoliation of malignant mesothelial cells. Similarly in advanced cases there is little, if any, exfoliation into fluid locules. However, effusions rich in malignant mesothelial cells can be present at any stage. Mesotheliomas of epithelial and mixed type shed cells either singly or in clumps, but cells from a mesothelioma of connective tissue type rarely exfoliate.

(a)i. Cytological characteristics of epithelial and mixed types

The cells may be present in tissue fragments, in cell groups or as isolated single cells. Effusions are often highly cellular, but in some cases exfoliation is poor. The fluid contains variable numbers of erythrocytes, lymphocytes, histiocytes and granulocytes. Exfoliation of malignant mesothelial cells on their own is rare.

Tissue fragments usually have a papillary or tubular structure. The former presents with a 'raspberry-like' appearance with nuclei situated away from the surface of the fragment. While this is a common feature of a mesothelioma, it is not specifically diagnostic. Paraffin sections of centrifuged cell deposits may contain tissue fragments showing histological evidence of diffuse malignant mesothelioma.

Malignant mesothelial cells presenting either singly or in groups show a wide variation in cell size but are, on average, larger than reactive mesothelial cells. There is usually minor increase in nuclear/ cytoplasmic ratio. The nuclei are round or oval, and are placed centrally or slightly off centre; binucleation is fairly common but multinucleation is rare. The nuclear outline appears smooth, or at most slightly wrinkled; the nuclear chromatin is coarsely granular and irregularly arranged. Nucleoli are large and single, or small and multiple but they are always characterized by sharp irregularities of outline. The cytoplasm is densely stained around the nucleus exaggerating the shading away effect at the periphery. This results in a finely vacuolated lace-like appearance. Large intra-cytoplasmic vacuoles are uncommon and when present they are due to degeneration or absorption of fluid.

ii. Cytological characteristics of connective tissue type

As exfoliation from this type of mesothelioma is rare cytology of effusions is not helpful. However, when these cells are present they are indistinguishable from connective tissue cells and are usually only recognized after review of histologically diagnosed cases.

(b) Special stains

These mainly comprise PAS and diastase–PAS in order to determine the presence or absence of mucin. The stains are best performed on paraffin sections, but may be used on smears. For details the reader is referred to the section of this chapter on histopathology.

(c) Diagnostic cytological criteria

The cells from a malignant mesothelioma should have the characteristics both of mesothelial cells and of malignancy, giving the immediate impression that they are 'atypical and of mesothelial origin'. Although this general rule is simple enough, the difficulties in differential diagnosis are frequent.

(d) Differential diagnosis

The cytological diagnosis of diffuse malignant mesothelioma depends on distinguishing malignant mesothelial cells from

   (i) reactive mesothelial cells,
   (ii) metastatic carcinoma.

(i) Reactive mesothelial cells

These can cause great diagnostic difficulties especially with effusions caused by infarction or cirrhosis. Pleomorphism can be marked and even 'raspberry' forms can be present. Correct diagnosis depends on the morphology of individual cells, with emphasis on the nuclear chromatin pattern. In reactive mesothelial cells this is dispersed, finely granular and regular. Nucleoli can be prominent and are often multiple, but they are round or oval without the sharp angularities seen in malignant cells. On the whole, cytoplasmic staining is less dense, but this feature is unreliable. Multinucleation is seen in reactive cells and the number of nuclei present is often greater than in malignant mesothelial cells. The appearance can imitate a foreign body giant cell.

(ii) Metastatic carcinoma

This is a commoner cause of serous effusions than diffuse malignant mesothelioma. In particular, difficulty may be experienced cytologically in distinguishing the following from mesothelioma.

(1) *Carcinoma of breast.* Exfoliation can occur as tissue fragments which superficially resemble the 'raspberry' forms of mesothelioma. However carcinomas show either acinar forms or solid tumour fragments, and the outline is smooth with nuclei placed at the outer edge of the fragment. In addition, individual cells show a higher nuclear/cytoplasmic ratio than malignant mesothelial cells.

(2) *Adenocarcinoma of lung.* Well-differentiated adenocarcinoma may be indistinguishable on cytological criteria when it is not possible to demonstrate mucin secretion. The cells and nuclei are rather large and the nucleoli more prominent.

(3) *Serous adenocarcinoma of ovary.* This presents difficulties both when exfoliation is in the form of papillary fragments and also in cases where this type of tumour exfoliates as single cells. In the latter type, cells usually show a higher nuclear/cytoplasmic ratio and there is more irregularity of nuclear outline.

(4) *Poorly differentiated squamous cell carcinoma.* These tumors exfoliate in a single cell form and are distinguished by a harder cytoplasmic outline, which sometimes shows a looped effect. In addition there is greater irregularity of nuclear form.

Cytology of aspirates and imprints

The cytology of both fine needle aspirates and imprints have the same morphological and staining properties. The fine needle aspiration biopsy may be useful in establishing a diagnosis of malignancy if a biopsy is not desirable.

The imprints are a valuable supplement to the diagnosis on frozen sections by giving more details of the cellular content. This is especially helpful in the connective tissue type and in the mixed type of malignant mesothelioma. The cytological criteria and differential diagnostic problems are the same as those encountered in effusions.

References

Berge, T. and Grontoft, O. (1965). Cytologic diagnosis of malignant pleural mesothelioma. *Acta Cytol.*, **9.**, 207–212

Butler, E.B. and Berry, A.V. (1974). Diffuse mesotheliomas: diagnostic criteria using exfoliative cytology. In Bogovski, P., Gilson, J.C., Timbrell, V. and Wagner, J.C. (eds.). *Biological Effects of Asbestos.* pp. 68–73. (Lyon: IARC Scientific Publications)

Dekker, A. and Bupp, P.A. (1978). Cytology of serous effusions. An investigation into the usefulness of cell blocks versus smears. *Am. J. Clin. Pathol.*, **70**, 855–860

Klempman, S. (1962). The exfoliative cytology of diffuse pleural mesotheliomas. *Cancer*, **15**, 691–704

Naylor, P. (1963). The exfoliative cytology of diffuse malignant mesothelioma. *J. Pathol. Bacteriol.*, **86**, 293–298

Spriggs, A.I. and Grunze, H. (1983) An unusual cytologic presentation of mesothelioma in serous effusions. *Acta Cytol.* **7** (3), 288–292

Warthin, A.S. (1897). The diagnosis of a primary sarcoma of the pleura from cells found in the pleural exudate. *Med. News (New York)*, **71**, 489–494

IV. CLINICAL FEATURES AND NATURAL HISTORY

(a) Symptoms and signs

Mesothelioma of pleura

The clinical features will depend on the stage that the disease has reached by the time the patient is examined. Initially there may be no symptoms at all, even though the tumour is already visible on radiological examination. The most common presenting symptom is a persistent pain in the chest which starts as a dull ache, and later it develops into a constant pain which may interfere with sleep. It usually involves the lateral chest wall of the affected side but may radiate to the back, to the shoulder or to the abdomen. The early symptoms are due to infiltration of the chest wall by tumour rather than to friction between the pleural surfaces, and therefore the character of the pain is different from that of pleurisy. A persistent pleural effusion often develops early in the course of the disease and the associated breathlessness due to compression of the lungs may be the presenting feature in some cases. This symptom can be present even though the tumour is relatively small. The effusion may become blood-stained, and although profuse at certain stages, the fluid usually diminishes as the pleural space becomes progressively obliterated due to the diffuse spread of the tumour. Cytological examination can be helpful in establishing the diagnosis. Cough, lassitude and weight loss may have been added to the list of symptoms by the time the patients present themselves for medical advice. Diminished chest movement may be observed due either to a pleural effusion, or to spread of tumour on the pleural surface, particularly if the costo-phrenic angle is involved. At an early stage the erythroid sedimentation rate may be raised and there is often a polymorph leucocytosis.

By the time the disease is firmly established there may be finger-clubbing. In late stages the movement of the chest may be limited due to the splinting of the chest wall by diffusely spreading tumour. There may be contraction and elevation of the diaphragm which becomes rigid with tumour. Symptoms of heart failure may become evident if there is spread of tumour to the pericardium. Symptoms may develop at other sites if the tumour has spread to other body cavities, such as the contra-lateral pleural or abdominal cavity.

Mesothelioma of peritoneum

Throughout all stages of the disease mesothelioma of the peritoneum does not have any particular feature which distinguishes it from other diffusely spreading intra-abdominal tumours. The presenting symptoms of mesothelioma of the peritoneum are even less specific than those of the pleural tumour. The initial symptom is usually a dull pain in the abdomen followed by abdominal swelling, loss of appetite and weight loss.

On examination large amounts of ascitic fluid may be present. This may initially be straw-coloured but later, blood-stained. The quantity of ascitic fluid diminishes as more of the peritoneal cavity becomes occupied by tumour. Locules of fluid may remain in the non-fused areas. A hard mass may be palpable as the tumour spreads, and a rigid tumour may be felt on rectal examination if the pelvic peritoneum is involved. Colicky pain and vomiting may be experienced by the patient as loops of bowel become adherent due to spread of the serosal tumour. Intestinal obstruction may not occur until quite late in the disease as only the outer layers of the gastrointestinal tract are invaded by tumour.

Mesothelioma of pericardium

The main feature is symptoms of increasing heart failure with dyspnoea, cardiac enlargement, tachycardia and liver enlargement, often erroneously attributed to ischaemic heart disease. The electrocardiogram typically shows a progressive low voltage pattern.

(b) Radiological features

Mesothelioma of pleura

The earliest radiological changes usually occur at the costo-phrenic angle. These may be due to small effusions, pleural thickening, or both. In addition there may be radiological signs of pleural plaques in the classical distribution along the lines of the lower ribs and on the central tendons of the diaphragm. These are particularly evident if calcification has occurred within the plaques.

In a proportion of cases of mesothelioma there may also be shadowing, particularly in the basal segments of the lungs, due to co-existing asbestosis. At a later stage, as the pleural thickening becomes more generalized, nodular shadows in the lung periphery may be visible if the pleural tumour has extended locally into the lung parenchyma. Screening of the patient may show diminished movement of the affected side of the chest with limitation of diaphragmatic excursion due to the rigidity caused by the diffuse spread of neoplasm. Enlargement of the mediastinum may become apparent as tumour spreads to the lymph nodes.

Mesothelioma of peritoneum

The radiological changes in peritoneal mesothelioma are not specific. Thickened zones of peritoneal tumour and/or ascites may be seen on plain x-ray examination, or by using ultra-sound techniques. In the later stages of the disease signs of intestinal obstruction will be evident. Chest x-ray showing evidence of pleural plaques and/or asbestosis may be diagnostically helpful.

Mesothelioma of pericardium

Enlargement often mimicking a simple effusion is the major radiological sign.

CT scanning

CT scanning has proved useful in providing a more exact outlining of the tumour in all sites.

(c) Aetiology

(i) Relation to fibrous minerals

In 85–90% of cases of diffuse malignant mesothelioma there is a history of exposure to fibrous minerals, the commonest being asbestos. In order for the fibrous particles to be potentially harmful, they must be released into the air and be small enough to be respirable. The ability to cause mesotheliomas in humans seems to depend on the physical properties of the fibres, and the degree of carcinogenicity is related to the proportion of fibres with diameters of

0.5–2.5 μm, and with lengths of 10–80 μm. If the fibres are curly, they tend to gyrate when breathed in, and this makes them liable to come into contact with the bronchial mucosa resulting in them being expectorated and then swallowed. On the other hand the straight needle-like fibres, because of their aerodynamic properties, are more likely to reach the periphery of the bronchial tree and here they enter the lung and pleural tissues either by direct penetration or by transportation within the lymphatic system, including movement into the inner thoracic wall.

Since most of the fibrous minerals are resistant to destruction, the majority remain in the tissues throughout the rest of the patients' lives. Data so far available indicates that the risk of mesothelioma increases with increasing amount of inhaled fibrous particles, i.e. there is a dose-response relationship.

The mineral fibres which have been implicated in the causation of mesotheliomas are in order of risk:

(1) *zeolite*   (a fibrous erionite)
(2) *crocidolite* (blue asbestos)
(3) *amosite*   (brown asbestos)
(4) *chrysotile*   (white asbestos)

Another type of asbestos, *tremolite*, which is not used commercially to any great extent, is sometimes found as an impurity with *chrysotile*. Cases of mesothelioma have followed exposure to fine-diameter fibres of *tremolite*, but not to the coarser type of this fibre. A further type of asbestos – *anthophyllite* – no longer used commercially, has not caused mesotheliomas.

(ii) Latent interval

There is a characteristically long latent interval between the time of first exposure to mineral fibres and the development of meso-thelioma. In most cases this interval varies between 25 and 40 years, but examples shorter than 10 years and longer than 60 years have been described.

(iii) Other causes

Small numbers of peritoneal mesotheliomas have been reported following radiotherapy for other malignant conditions with latent intervals of 7–16 years.

A single case of peritoneal mesothelioma occurred 36 years after cholangiography with thorotrast.

(iv) Unknown

In approximately 10–15% of cases of mesothelioma there is no known contact with mineral fibres or with any other potential carcinogenic agent. There is no evidence to suggest that cigarette smoking has any influence on the development of mesothelioma.

(d) Epidemiology

(i) Geographical distribution

As there is such a close correlation between the exposure to certain mineral fibres and the development of mesotheliomas, the tumour is most commonly found where these fibres are mined or used in manufacturing processes, in installations and during demolition processes. The development of mesothelioma also depends on the type and size of mineral fibres.

The information on the geographical distribution of mesotheliomas is at present incomplete, and because of changes in laws and in working practices, there will inevitably be a change in the future pattern of distribution.

Mining areas. In two villages in Turkey, where an erionite-type mineral (zeolite) is found, and is extensively used locally in the building of houses, a high incidence of mesotheliomas is recorded in the local inhabitants. This mineral has a fine diameter fibre. Mesotheliomas have been reported in Western India and there is a possible association with zeolite in this area. Although zeolite is generally widely distributed around the world the only other known sites with comparably fine diameter fibres are in Oregon, USA and in New Zealand. No mesotheliomas have been reported in these two sites, but they are now the subject of prospective epidemiological studies.

In South Africa two types of crocidolite asbestos are mined – one in the northern part of Cape Province (Cape Blue), which has extremely fine diameter fibres ranging from 0.09 to 0.8 μm; the other in the Transvaal (Transvaal Blue) with a coarser diameter of fibre ranging from 0.2 to 2.5 μm. Amosite asbestos mines are situated in the South, near the Swaziland border. Of 88 cases of mesothelioma reported from these mining areas, 83 worked with Cape Blue crocidolite, 4 with amosite, 1 with Transvaal Blue crocidolite, but none were reported in the chrysotile mines.

In Wittenoom, Western Australia, where fine diameter crocidolite was mined, 26 cases of mesothelioma have occurred in a work force of 6200 men, many of whom have not yet been traced.

By contrast only eleven cases of mesothelioma have occurred in a work force of 11 379 chrysotile miners and millers in Quebec. Two of these had also been exposed to crocidolite. Only one case of mesothelioma has been found in the chrysotile mining and milling plant in Balangero, Northern Italy, and none in the Rhodesian chrysotile mines.

Information on the frequency of mesothelioma in the chrysotile mines in the USSR is not available.

The distribution of mesotheliomas associated with the amphibole tremolite seems to depend on the fibre dimensions of the mineral at the various locations. In California where it has a flaky consistency, no disease has been reported. In Quebec, where it is mined in conjunction with chrysotile in certain deposits, the fibre diameter is more than 1.0 μm. In New York State a few cases of mesothelioma have been recorded in association with the finer diameter fibres of tremolite, but most of this mineral which is found amongst the talc deposits, is of a coarser type. In the population around the asbestos mines in Cyprus, a few mesotheliomas have been noted. These deposits which are predominantly of chrysotile type also contain fine diameter fibres of tremolite. Coarse-fibre tremolite in the rural areas of Czechoslovakia, Yugoslavia, Bulgaria and Greece has not caused tumours. The finest type of tremolite is mined in South Korea, and following the high number of mesotheliomas in this locality production of this type of asbestos has now been stopped.

Industrial areas. With regard to the geographical distribution of mesotheliomas in relation to industrial workers, the pattern reflects the centres where asbestos has been used extensively, over a period of time. Clusters of cases of mesothelioma are consistently found in those cities and towns where ship-building is a major industry. Cases have also occurred in those cities and towns where there are factories using asbestos, particularly crocidolite and to a lesser extent amosite. Mesotheliomas occur in workers in the thermal insulation industry and also in building and demolition industries. Since these occupations are practised in most major cities and towns, there are few places where the tumour does not occur.

Examples of factory populations exposed to a single type of fibre are rare, as most industrial processes have involved mixtures of different fibres. A cohort of workers in England who manufactured military gas mask filters during the second world war were exclusively exposed to crocidolite. Thirty-nine mesotheliomas in a work force of 1600 have been reported from this factory, and clusters of mesotheliomas have occurred in other towns where the military gas masks were made, both in England and in Canada. In a factory which manufactured civilian gas masks, where the majority of workers were exclusively exposed to chrysotile, only one mesothelioma in a workforce of 570 has been reported, and that worker probably had also assembled military gas masks in another factory, and had therefore also been exposed to crocidolite.

(ii) Age and sex distribution

In those people whose mesotheliomas are related to mineral fibre exposure, two age groups can be defined. They relate (1) to those who have been *environmentally* exposed to mineral fibres since birth – they tend to develop mesotheliomas in the 45–50 year age group and (2) to those who have been *occupationally* exposed to asbestos or other fibrous minerals. When the initial contact is not made until they are 20 years of age, or more, they tend to develop mesotheliomas in the 60–70 year age group.

Amongst those people whose mesotheliomas are not related to mineral fibre exposure is a small group of children, the youngest being 1½ years of age.

The sex distribution of mesotheliomas is in keeping with the experience of mineral fibre exposure. In the mining communes both males and females may be affected because of environmental exposure to fibres, but the majority of tumours occur in the males who are also occupationally exposed.

In many facturing industries there is a predominance of mesotheliomas in males because this reflects the sex ratio of the workforce generally at risk. However where fibre exposure has occurred in factories in which there is a predominance of women, the

mesotheliomas have occurred in a predominantly female distribution. For example, in the wartime gas mask factory referred to
previously, only a few men were employed out of a total workforce
of 1600. To date only one mesothelioma has occurred in the male
workers, but 38 in the females.

(iii) Frequency

A major problem in establishing the frequency with which mesothelioma occurs is inherent in the difficulty of making a confident
diagnosis of the tumour. Until recent years this neoplasm was not
generally recognized by pathologists as being a separate entity. Most
cases of pleural and peritoneal mesothelioma were wrongly labelled
'metastatic tumour from an unknown primary source'. From about
1960 onwards however, the clinical, radiological and pathological
criteria have been more clearly defined. With an increasing aware-
ness of the condition, more accurate diagnoses of mesothelioma
were made.

The frequency with which mesothelioma occurs depends on the
population that is being sampled. In general terms it is a rare
tumour. In the Malmö series of consecutive autopsies the incidence
of pleural mesothelioma in females was 0.1% and in males 0.3%.
The incidence of peritoneal mesotheliomas in males and females was
0.1%. In the United Kingdom during the year 1968 there was a total
of 153 cases of mesothelioma recorded by death certification. In
each succeeding year however the number has increased, and while
this may be attributable in part to more reliable diagnosis, the trend
of almost doubling the number of cases within a decade to 292 cases
per year by 1976 indicates that the increase is real.

Though the number of mesotheliomas within the general population is small, the frequency with which it occurs in those who have
worked with asbestos underlines the risk of this form of exposure.
Insulators and laggers carry the highest risk – between 6% and 9%
dying from mesothelioma.

(e) Prognosis

The period from the presenting symptoms of mesothelioma to death
is usually of the order of 18 months to 2 years, but occasionally a

patient may survive a period of 5 years or so. It is not known when the tumour process starts within the long latent interval. Some cases have been reported in which a mesothelioma has been incidentally diagnosed before symptoms were present. In these cases an apparently longer survival time is suggested. The outcome of the disease is uninfluenced by the treatment which is currently available.

References

Acheson, E.D., Gardner, M.J., Pippard, E.C. and Grime, L.P. (1982). Mortality of two groups of women who manufactured gas masks from chrysotile and crocidolite asbestos: a 40-year follow-up. *Brit.J.Ind.Med.*, **39**, 344–348

Aisner, J. and Wiernik, P.H. (1978). Malignant mesothelioma. Current status and future prospects. *Chest*, **74**, No. 4, 438–444

Antman, K.H. (1980). Current concepts. Malignant mesothelioma. *N. Engl. J. Med.*, **303**, 200–202

Antman, K.H., Corson, J.M., Li, F.P., Greenberger, J., Sytkowski, A., Henson, D.E. and Weinstein, L. (1983). Malignant mesothelioma following radiation exposure. *J.Clin.Oncol.*, **1**, (11), 695–700

Artvinli, M. and Baris, Y.I. (1982). Environmental fiber-induced pleura-pulmonary diseases in an Anatolian village. *Arch.Environ. Health*, **37**, 177–181

Babcock, T.L., Powell, D.H. and Bothwell, R.S. (1976). Radiation-induced peritoneal mesothelioma. *J.Surg.Oncol.* **8**, 369–372

Baris, Y.I., Simonato, L., Saracci, R., Skidmore, J.W. and Artvinli, M. (1981). Malignant mesothelioma and radiological chest abnormalities in two villages in central Turkey. *Lancet*, **1**, 984–987

Becklake, M.R., (1982). Asbestos-related diseases of the lung and pleura. *Am.Rev.Resp.Dis.*, **126**, 187–194

Berge, T. and Lundberg, S. (1977). Cancer in Malmö, 1958–1969. An autopsy study. *Acta Pathol. Microbiol. Scand. Section A.*, Suppl. **260**, 128–133 and 142–143

Boman, G., Schubert, V., Svane, B., Westerholm, P., Bolinder, E., Rohl, A.N. and Fischbein, A. (1982). Malignant mesothelioma in Turkish immigrants residing in Sweden. *Scand.J. Work Environ. Health*, **8**, 108–112

Brenner, J., Sordillo, P.P. and Magill, G.B. (1981). Malignant mesothelioma in children: report of seven cases and review of the literature. *Med.Pediatr. Oncol.* **9**, 367–373

Brenner, J., Sordillo, P.P., Magill, G.B. and Golbey, R.B. (1982). Malignant mesothelioma of the pleura. Review of 123 patients. *Cancer*, **49**, 2431–2435

Chahinian, A.P. (1982). Malignant mesothelioma. In: Greenspan, E.M. (Ed.). *Clinical Interpretation and Practice of Cancer Chemotherapy.* Chapter 26, pp. 599–606. (New York: Raven Press)

Churg, A., Warnock, M.L. and Bensch, K.G. (1978). Malignant mesothelioma arising after direct application of asbestos and fiber glass to the pericardium. *Am.Rev.Resp.Dis.*, **118**, 419–424

Clemmesen. J. and Hjalgrim-Jensen, S. (1981). Cancer incidence among 5686 asbestos-cement workers followed from 1943 through 1976. *Ecotoxicol.Environ.Safety*, **51**, 15–23

Cochrane, J.C. and Webster I. (1978). Mesothelioma in relation to asbestos fibre exposure. A review of 70 serial cases. *S.A.Med. J.*, 279–281

Craighead, J.E. and Mossman, B.T. (1982). The pathogenesis of asbestos-associated diseases. *N.Engl.J.Med.*, **306**, 1446–1455

Dunhill, M.S. (1984). Pleural mesothelioma. Editorial. *Eur.J.Respir.Dis.*, **65**, 159–161

Elmes, P.C. and Simpson, M.J.C. (1976). The clinical aspects of mesothelioma. *Q. J.Med.*, **XLV**, No. 179, 427–449

Gardner, M.J., Acheson, E.D. and Winter, P.D. (1982). Mortality from mesothelioma of the pleura during 1968–78 in England and Wales. *Br.J.Cancer*, **46**, 81–88

Gardner, M.J., Winter, P.D. and Acheson, E.D. (1982). Variation in cancer mortality among local authority areas in England and Wales: relations with environmental factors and search for causes. *Br.Med.J.*, **284**, 784–787

Glickman, L.T., Domanski, L.M., Maguire, T.G., Dubielzig, R.R. and Churg, A. (1983). Mesothelioma in pet dogs associated with exposure of their owners to asbestos. *Environ. Res.*, **32**, 305–313

Harington, J.S. (1981). Fiber carcinogenesis. Epidemiologic observations and the Stanton hypothesis. *J.Natl. Cancer Inst.*, **67**, No.5, 977–989

Harrison, R.N. (1984). Sarcomatous pleural mesothelioma and cerebral metastases: case report and a review of eight cases. *Eur.J.Respir.Dis.*, **65**, 185–188

Hirsch, A., Brochard, P., De Cremoux, H., Erkan, L., Sébastien, P., Di Menza, L. and Bignon, J. (1982). Features of asbestos-exposed and unexposed mesothelioma. *Am.J.Ind.Med.*, **3**, 413–422

Jones, J.S.P., Pooley, F.D., Sawle, G.W., Madeley, R.J., Smith, P.G., Berry, G., Wignall, B.K. and Aggarwal, A. (1980). The consequences of exposure to asbestos dust in a wartime gas mask factory. In Wagner, J.C. (ed.). *Biological Effects of Mineral Fibres*. pp. 637–653. (IARC Scientific Publications No. 30. INSERM Symposia Series, Vol. 92). (Lyon)

Kagan, E., and Jacobson, J. (1983). Lymphoid and plasma cell malignancies; asbestos-related disorders of long latency. *Am.J.Clin.Pathol.*, **80**, 14–20

Kahn, E.I., Rohl, A., Barrett, E.W. and Suzuki, Y. (1980). Primary pericardial mesothelioma following exposure to asbestos. *Environ. Res.*, **23**, 270–281

Lajartre, M.D., Cornet, E., Corroller, J., Moigneteau, Ch.R., Dupon, H., Rembeaux, A., Michaud, J.L., Charritte, A. and Gugelot, A. (1976). Étude clinique et professionelle de 54 mésothéliomes pleuraux diffus. *Rev.Fr.Mal.Resp.*, Suppl. 2, **4**, 63–74

Law, M.R., Gregor, A., Hudson, M.E., Bloom, H.J.G. and Turner-Warwick, M. (1984). Malignant mesothelioma of the pleura: a study of 52 treated and 64 untreated patients. *Thorax*, **39**, 255–259

Law, M.R., Hudson, M.E. and Turner-Warwick, M. (1984). Malignant mesothelioma of the pleura: clinical aspects and symptomatic treatment. *Eur.J.Respir.Dis.*, **65**, 162–168

McDonald, A.D. and Fry, J.S. (1982). Mesothelioma and fiber type in three American asbestos factories – a preliminary report. *Scand.J.Work Environ.Health*, **8**, suppl. 1, 53–58

McDonald, J.C. and McDonald, A.D. (1977). Epidemiology of mesothelioma from estimated incidence. *Prev.Med.*, **6**, 426–446

Mårtensson, G., Hagmar, B. and Zettergren, L. (1984). Diagnosis and prognosis in malignant pleural mesothelioma: a prospective study. *Eur.J.Respir.Dis.*, **65**, 169–178

Mårtensson, G., Larsson, S. and Zettergren, L. (1984). Malignant mesothelioma in two pairs of siblings: is there a hereditary predisposing factor? *Eur.J.Respir.Dis.*, **65,** 179–184

Maurer, R. and Egloff, B. (1975). Malignant peritoneal mesothelioma after cholangiography with Thorotrast. *Cancer*, **36,** 1381–1385

Newhouse, M.L. (1981). Epidemiology of asbestos-related tumors. *Seminars Oncol.*, **8,** No. 3, 250–257

Newhouse, M.L. and Berry, G. (1976). Predictions of mortality from mesothelial tumours in asbestos factory workers. *Br.J.Ind.Med.*, **33,** 147–151

Pelnar, P.V. (1983). Non-asbestos related malignant mesothelioma. A review of the scientific and medical literature. Canadian Asbestos Information Centre, Montreal, P.Q., Canada

Rubino, G.F., Piolatto, G., Newhouse, M.L., Scansetti, G., Aresini, G.A. and Murray, R. (1979). Mortality of chrysotile asbestos workers at the Balangero Mine, Northern Italy. *Br.J.Ind.Med.*, **36,** 187–194

Stanton, M.F., Layard, M., Tegeris, A., Miller, E., May, M., Morgan, E. and Smith, A.(1981). Relation of particle dimension to carcinogenicity in amphibole asbestoses and other fibrous minerals. *J.Natl.Cancer Inst.*, **67,** 965–975

Stock, R.J., Fu, Y.S. and Carter, J.R. (1979). Malignant peritoneal mesothelioma following radiotherapy for seminoma of the testis. *Cancer*, **44,** 914–919

Wagner J.C. (1980). Environmental and occupational exposure to natural mineral fibres. In Wagner, J.C. (ed.). *Biological Effects of Mineral Fibres.* pp. 995–997. (IARC Scientific Publications No. 30, INSERM Symposia Series Vol. 92). (Lyon)

Wagner, J.C., Sleggs, C.A. and Marchand, P. (1960). Diffuse pleural mesothelioma and asbestos exposure in the Northwestern Cape Province. *Br.J.Ind.Med.*, **17,** 260–271

Whitwell, F., Scott, J. and Grimshaw, M. (1977). Relationship between occupations and asbestos fibre content of the lungs in patients with pleural mesothelioma, lung cancer and other diseases. *Thorax*, **32,** 377–386

Yaziciolgu, S., Ilcayto, R., Balci, K., Sayli, B.S. and Yorulmaz, B. (1980). Pleural calcification, pleural mesotheliomas and bronchial cancers caused by tremolite dust. *Thorax*, **35,** 564–569

Zielhuis, R.L. (1977). *Public Health Risks of Exposure to Asbestos.* Commission of the European Communities. (Oxford: Pergamon Press)

V. MESOTHELIOMA PANELS

The highly variable appearance in the histopathological picture of mesothelioma, its very low frequency in many geographical areas and the legal consequences of this tumour in some countries have led to the establishment of mesothelioma panels. Their aim is to reach agreement on the pathological diagnosis. The information is used for diagnostic and epidemiological studies and, in some countries for legal purposes.

Most panels consist of pathologists only, but some also have clinical and/or occupational health officers as members. The majority of panels are nationally based but some independent regional panels also exist. There is an international panel for the European Economic Community. (C.E.C. Mesothelioma Panel).

Some panels are permanent, while others have existed in order to undertake a specific project. The working arrangements for panels vary, but a satisfactory scheme usually evolves over a period of time, depending on the purpose of the individual panel and on local logistic requirements.

The organization of the panels may be very different, ranging from governmental, via semi-official to independent organizations. The methods of operation are also different. Some panels have meetings only; others circulate slides to panel members but do not have meetings, while others have panel meetings and a postal circulation of slides. It is acknowledged in mesothelioma panels that observer variations occur, but the more experience that is gained in examining this rare tumour, the greater is the diagnostic agreement.

Favourable conditions for the working of a panel are as follows.

(1) Circulation of slides to the members of the panel a few weeks before the meeting.

(2) Regular meetings in which cases are discussed, together with a review of old, doubtful cases.

(3) Use of a voting system, preferably written, in order to avoid the possibility of individual members influencing each other.

(4) Provision of additional data, including the clinical behaviour of the process, the gross pathological appearance and any available information on additional investigations, such as electron microscopy and histochemistry.

(5) A second vote by panel members taking into consideration all the additional information.

(6) The conclusion of the panel, preferably in the form of a definite diagnosis.

It is preferable that material is sent to the panel co-ordinator in the form of paraffin blocks. A haematoxylin and eosin stained slide and three unstained spare slides are then sent to each panel member together with a voting sheet. Clinical and occupational information can be included in a separate envelope to be opened after the pathologist has made the initial histological diagnosis. The results from each panel member are then returned to the co-ordinator who then informs all members of the various opinions.

Experience has shown that haematoxylin and eosin, and diastase–PAS-stained sections are usually sufficient for diagnostic purposes.

The voting systems used by many panels are very similar. The C.E.C. Mesothelioma Panel uses the following categories:

A. Definite malignant mesothelioma – no doubt as to the histopathological diagnosis.

B. Probable malignant mesothelioma – the reason for hesitation may be lack of material, bad quality, lack of differentiation, absence of certain histological details which give rise to slight doubt.

C. Possible malignant mesothelioma – the diagnosis cannot be denied but there is insufficient evidence to come to a positive conclusion.

D. Improbable malignant mesothelioma – probably not a mesothelioma but the diagnosis cannot be absolutely denied.

E. Definitely not a malignant mesothelioma.

In category E, the alternative diagnosis is suggested.

This scheme can be used not only by panels, but also by individual pathologists. When summarizing the results groups A and B can be taken together as positive, and groups D and E as negative, while group C remains doubtful. Groups A and B can be used as the basis for including cases in a mesothelioma register. The use of this voting system makes it possible to compare opinions of different observers and also of the same observers on different occasions. The use of this system in a panel usually leads to good or reasonable agreement between panel members. Second viewing of the slides after more experience usually increases agreement. As all panels may differ from each other in their procedures it may not be possible to compare exactly the results in relation to geographical distribution, frequency of different types and localization etc. Hopefully an agreed uniform approach to histological diagnosis may lead to these types of comparative studies becoming more relevant.

For futher information a list is supplied of all Mesothelioma Panels that we have traced, together with the names and addresses of the Chairman or the person who supplied the information.

Commission Of The European Communities (C.E.C.)

C.E.C. Mesothelioma Panel
c/o J.S.P. Jones
Department of Pathology
City Hospital
Nottingham NG5 1PB
England

Chairman: W.J. Hunter
Health and Safety Directorate
Directorate-General Employment, Social Affairs and Education
Commission of the European Communities
Bâtiment Jean Monnet
Plateau du Kirchberg
Luxembourg

Australia

The Royal College of Pathologists of Australasia
Mesothelioma Panel
Co-ordinator: T. Jelihovsky
Convenor of the Australian Mesothelioma Surveillance Program:
D. Ferguson
Commonwealth Institute of Health
Building A 27
University of Sydney
NSW Australia 2006

Belgium

c/o P. Balasse
Service d'Anatomie Pathologique
Hôpital Universitaire Erasme
808 Route de Lennick
1070 Bruxelles

Canada

Canadian Mesothelioma Panel
c/o Canadian Tumour Reference Centre
National Cancer Institute of Canada
c/o W.T.E. McCaughey
Clinical Studies Unit Building
Ottawa Civic Hospital
60 Ruskin Avenue
Ottawa
Canada K1Y 4M9

Denmark

c/o C. Lund
Patologisk Institut
Centralsygehuset i Holstebro
Laegaardvej 12
7500 Holstebro

Federal Republic of Germany

Mesotheliomregister des Hauptverbandes der gewerblichen
Berufsgenossenschaften Bonn
c/o H. Otto
Pathologisches Institut des Städtischen Kliniken
Beurhausstrasse 40
D-4600 Dortmund 1

France

French Mesothelioma Register/Registre Français des Mésothéliomes
c/o J. Bignon
Clinique de Pathologie Respiratoire

Centre Hospitalier Intercommunal
40, Avenue de Verdun
94010 Créteil

Ireland

c/o T.M. Healy
Department of Pathology
University College
Earlsfort Terrace
Dublin 2

Italy

Registro Italiano dei Mesoteliomi (R.M.I.)
c/o A. Donna
Servizio di Anatomia e Istologia Patologica
Ospedale Generale Provinciale
Via Venezia 18
15100 Alessandria

Panel Italiano dei Mesoteliomi
c/o A.M. Mancini
Istituto di Anatomia e Istologia Patologica
Policlinico S. Orsola – Università degli Studi
V. Masserenti
40138 Bologna

Netherlands

Dutch Mesothelioma Panel
c/o H.T. Planteydt
Streeklaboratorium 'Zeeland'
Molenwater 47
4331 SC Middelburg

Republic of South Africa

Mesothelioma Panel and Register
c/o I. Webster

National Centre for Occupational Health
P.O. Box 4788
Johannesburg 2000

Switzerland

c/o J.R. Rüttner
Institut für Pathologie der Universität Zürich
Universitätsspital
Schmelzbergstrasse 12
8091 Zurich

United Kingdom

c/o J.S.P. Jones
Department of Pathology
City Hospital
Nottingham NG5 1PB
or: J.C. Wagner
M.R.C. Pneumoconiosis Unit
Llandough Hospital
Penarth, South Glamorgan

United States of America

U.S. Mesothelioma Panel
Chairman: C. Carrington
             Department of Pathology
             Stanford University School of Medicine
             Palo Alto
             California

References

Bignon, J., Sébastien, P., di Menza, L., Nebut, M. et Payan, H. (1979). Registre Français des Mésothéliomes 1965–1978. *Rev.Fr.Mal.Resp.*, **7**, 223–242

Ferguson, D. and Ng,Th. (1980). Australian mesothelioma register. *Med.J.Austr.* **1**, 150–152

Greenberg, M. and Lloyd Davies, T.A. (1974). Mesothelioma register 1967–1968. *Br.J.Ind.Med.*, **31**, 91–104

Hunter, W.J. and Recht, P. (1980). Scientific aspects of the work of the Commission of the European Communities on asbestos. In Wagner, J.C. (ed.). *Biological Effects of Mineral Fibres*. pp. 775–782. (IARC Scientific Publications No. 30, INSERM Symposia Series, vol. 92) (Lyon)

Kannerstein, M. and Churg, J. (1979). Functions of mesothelioma panels. *Ann. N.Y.Acad.Sci.*, **330**, 433–439

McCaughey, W.T.E., Al-Jabi, M. and Kannerstein, M. (1980). A Canadian experience of the pathological diagnosis of diffuse mesothelioma. In Wagner, J.C. (ed.). *Biological Effects of Mineral Fibres*. pp. 207–210. (IARC Scientific Publications No. 30. INSERM Symposia Series Vol. 92) (Lyon)

McCaughey, W.T.E. and Oldham, P.D. (1973). Diffuse mesothelioma: observer variation in histological diagnosis. In Bogovski, P., Gilson, J.C., Timbrell, V. and Wagner, J.C. (eds). *Biological Effects of Asbestos*. pp. 58–61 (IARC Scientific Publications No. 8) (Lyon)

McDonald, A.D., Magner, D. and Eyssen, G. (1973). Primary malignant mesothelial tumours in Canada, 1960–1968. A pathologic review by the Mesothelioma Panel of the Canadian Tumour Reference Centre. *Cancer*, **31**, 869–876

Otto, H. (1980). Das berufsbedingte Mesotheliom in der B.R.D. *Pathologe*, **2**, 8–18

Planteydt, H.T. (1979). Netherlands mesothelioma register. *Ann.N.Y.Acad.Sci.* **330**, 467–472

Planteydt, H.T. (1980). Experiences with observer variation in mesothelioma panels. In Wagner, J.C. (ed.). *Biological Effects of Mineral Fibres*. pp. 211–216. (IARC Scientific Publications No. 30, INSERM Symposia Series Vol. 92) (Lyon)

VI. THEORIES ON THE PATHOGENESIS OF MESOTHELIOMA

(a) Morphological concept

The characteristic morphological features of a mesothelioma are in accordance with the cellular properties of the mesothelium. These are neoplastic changes of epithelial type or of connective tissue type, or more commonly, a combination of both. For this reason most tumours are of mixed type but may show a bias towards one or other extremes and special differentiation into several connective tissue elements as indicated in the diagram (Figure 3).

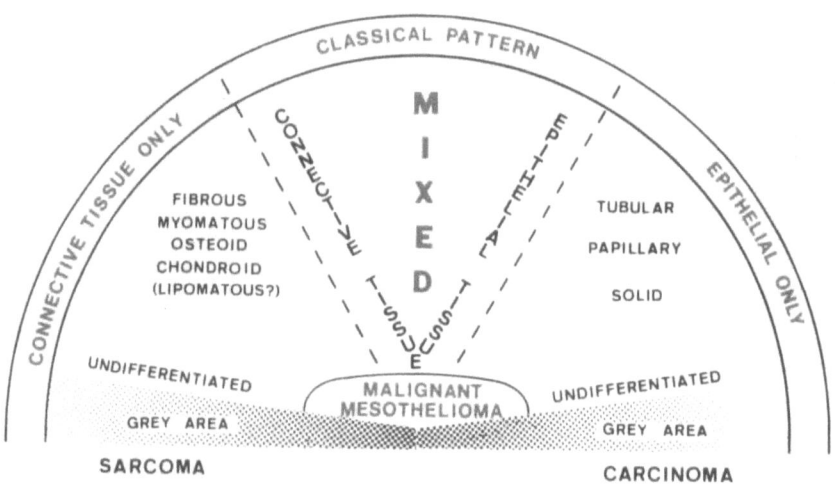

Figure 3 Spectrum of the differentiation of diffuse malignant mesothelioma according to the morphological concept

(b) Embryological concept

The so-called *Mesodermoma concept* proposed by Donna and Pravano (1977) and modified by Donna and Betta (1981) is an embryological approach to primary tumours of the coelomic surfaces with the emphasis on the mesothelium being of mesodermal origin. The following classification summarizes the concept of mesodermoma:

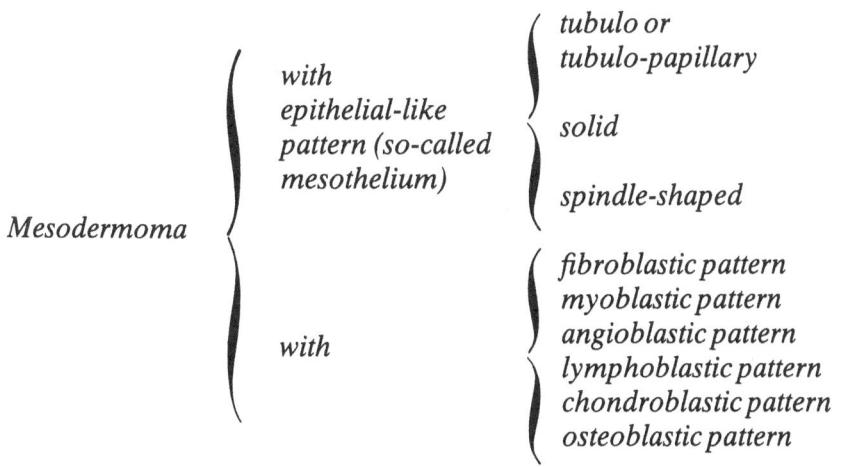

This embryological approach strongly supports the multipotential property of mesothelial cells to differentiate along diverse cell lines and it indicates the wide range of differential activity. In the opinion of the proposers of this concept, transition to epithelial-like cells, resembling mesoderm of coelomic surfaces, must always be found in order to make a histological diagnosis of mesodermoma.

The embryologically based concept only outdistances the content of this atlas by introducing the word *Mesodermoma* and by suggesting lines of differentiation into vascular and lymphoblastic tumours. The hypothesis provides an interesting possible explanation for the pathogenesis of this unique tumour group.

References

Donna, A. and Betta, P.G. (1981). Mesodermomas; a new embryological approach to primary tumours of coelomic surfaces. *Histopathology*, **5**, 31–44

Donna, A. and Provana, A. (1977). Considerations and proposals about mesotheliomas based on their morphological appearances. *Pathologica*, **69**, 441–468

VII. DIAGNOSTIC DEVELOPMENTS

(a) Electron microscopy

Among the ultrastructural features of a mesothelioma the following are commonly found.

(1) Large, irregular indented nucleus.
(2) Desmosomes.
(3) Thickened basal lamina.
(4) Numerous long and slender microvilli.
(5) Numerous intracytoplasmic filaments.

Transmission electron microscopy has been found to be of some value, while scanning electron microscopy is of no value in diagnosing mesothelioma.

References

Bolen, J.W. and Thorning, D. (1980). Mesotheliomas. A light-and electron-microscopical study concerning histogenetic relationships between the epithelial and the mesenchymal variants. *Am.J.Surg.Pathol.* **4** (5), 451–464

Butler, E.B. and Johnson, N.F. (1980). The use of electron microscopy in the diagnosis of diffuse mesothelioma using human pleural effusions. In Wagner, J.C. (ed.). *Biological Effects of Mineral Fibres*. pp. 409–418. (IARC Scientific Publications No. 30. INSERM Symposia Series Vol. 92) (Lyon)

Dardick, I., Srigley, J.R., McCaughey, W.T.E., van Nostrand, A.W.P., and Ritchie, A.C. (1984). Ultra structural aspects of the histogenesis of diffuse and localised mesothelioma. *Virch.Arch.(Pathol.Anat.)*, **402**, 373–388

Mather, J., Stanbridge, C.M. and Butler, E.B. (1981). Method for the removal of selected cells from cytology smear preparations for transmission electron microscopy. *J.Clin.Pathol.* **34**, 1355–1357

Stoebner, P. and Brambilla, E. (1982). Ultrastructural diagnosis of pleural tumours. *Pathol. Res.Pract.*, **173**, 402–416

Suzuki, Y. (1981). Pathology of human malignant mesothelioma. *Semin. Oncol.*, **8**, No. 3, 268–282

Suzuki, Y., Churg, J. and Kannerstein, M. (1976). Ultrastructure of human malignant diffuse mesothelioma. *Am.J.Pathol.*, **85**, 241–262

Warhol, M.J., Hickey, W.F. and Corson, J.M. (1982). Malignant mesothelioma – ultrastructural distinction from adenocarcinoma. *Am.J.Surg.Pathol.*, **6**, 307–314

(b) Special staining

Apart from the stains mentioned previously (see page 14), special stains are not very helpful. However, a technique developed by Donna *et al.* (1980) indicates the possibility of identification of neoplastic mesothelial cells from reactive mesothelial cells and distinguishes them from mucin-secreting cells in serous effusions.

References

Donna, A., Betta, P.G., Gagliardi, F. and Provana, A. (1980). A new method for detecting activated and neoplastic mesothelial cells in serous effusions. In Wagner, J.C. (ed.). *Biological Effects of Mineral Fibres.* pp. 183–186. (IARC Scientific Publications No. 30, INSERM Symposia Series Vol. 92) (Lyon)

Donna, A., Betta, P.G., Provana, A. and Gagliardi, F. (1980). A cytoplasmic distinctive feature of activated and neoplastic mesothelial cells at phase contrast microscopy. *Pathologica,* **72,** 279–285

(c) Immunopathology

The elaborate modern techniques of purifying specific antigens as cell markers may prove to be useful in the diagnosis of mesothelioma.

Immunofluorescent staining using antisera against reactive as well as neoplastic mesothelial cells has recently been reported.

Carcinoembryonic antigen (CEA) is reported to be absent in diffuse malignant mesothelioma, but to be present in bronchiolo-alveolar cell carcinoma and other adenocarcinomas.

Ca 1 antibody has been found in an immuno-cytochemical procedure on smears of cells from two mesotheliomas but not in reactive mesothelioma cells.

These antibodies were also demonstrated in other malignant tumours, but the significance of the result of this method has been questioned.

In recent investigations it is claimed that mesotheliomas reveal immunologic staining for 63 kd keratin, which might be helpful in differentiating mesothelioma from adenocarcinoma. Less specific keratins are also reported in other investigated cases of mesothelioma.

References

Corson, J.M. and Pinkus, G.S. (1982). Mesothelioma: Profile of keratin proteins and carcinoembryonic antigen. *Am.J.Pathol.,* **108,** 80–87

Herbert, A. and Gallagher, P.J. (1982). Interpretation of pleural biopsy specimens and aspirates with the immunoperoxidase technique. *Thorax, 37*, 822–827

Holden, J. and Churg, A. (1984). Immunohistochemical staining for keratin and carcinoembryonic antigen in the diagnosis of malignant mesothelioma. *Am.J.Surg.Pathol.*, **8**, 277–279

Said, J.W. (1983). Immunohistochemical localization of keratin proteins in tumour diagnosis. *Hum.Pathol.*, **14**, 1017–1019

Singh, G., Dekker, A. and Whiteside, T.L. (1979). Anti-mesothelial cell serum: a diagnostic reagent for malignant mesothelioma. *Fed.Proc.*, **38**, 912

Wang, N.S., Huang, S.N. and Gold, P. (1979). Absence of carcinoembryonic antigen-like material in mesothelioma. *Cancer*, **44**, 937–943

Wang, N.S., Huang, S.N. and Gold, P. (1979). Carcinoembryonic antigen (C.E.A.)-like material in mesothelioma and other lung cancers. *Lab. Invest.*, **4**, 291

Whitaker, D. and Shilkin, K.B. (1981). Carcinoembryonic antigen in tissue diagnosis of malignant mesothelioma. *Lancet*, **1**, 1369

Whitaker, D., Sterrett, G.F. and Shilkin, K.B. (1982). Detection of tissue CEA-like substance as an aid in the differential diagnosis of malignant mesothelioma. *Pathology*, **14**, 255–258

Woods, J.C., Spriggs, A.I., Harris, H. and McGee, J.O'D. (1982). A new marker for human cancer cells. 3. Immunocytochemical detection of malignant cells in serous fluids with the Ca 1 antibody. *Lancet*, **2**, 512–514

(d) Morphometry and cytophotometry

In pleural effusions mesothelioma cells have a greater mean nuclear area and mean cytoplasmic area than reactive mesothelial cells. Comparing the cells of pleural mesothelioma with those of peritoneal mesothelioma the first have larger nuclei, a more pronounced anisokaryosis and a higher nuclear-cytoplasmic ratio. This is thought to be due to more extensive vacuolisation in peritoneal mesothelioma. By this method mesothelioma and metastases from other tumours cannot be distinguished.

Flow-cytometric analyses of the DNA content and behaviour with regard to ploidism have been performed, but so far without convincing results.

References

Alons, C.L., Veldhuizen, R.W. and Boon, M.E. (1981). Learning from quantitation. *Anal.Quant.Cytol.*, **3**, 178–181

Boon, M.E., Posthuma, H.S., Ruiter, D.J. and van Andel, J.G. (1981). Secreting peritoneal mesothelioma. Report of a case with cytological, ultrastructural, morphometric and histological studies. *Virch.Arch.Abt.A.Pathol. Anat.*, **392**, 33–44

Isoda, K., and Hamamoto, Y. (1983). Polypoid mesothelial cells in pleural fluid. *Acta Pathol. Jpn.*, **33**, (4), 733–738

Isoda, K., Sobajima, T., Kin, H., Fukuda, H. and Hamamoto, Y. (1983). A consideration on histopathologic variability of diffuse pleural mesothelioma based on DNA cytophotometry. *Acta Pathol. Jpn.*, **33** (4), 807–816

Kwee, W.S. (1982). Quantitative and qualitative studies of malignant mesothelioma. *Thesis*, Amsterdam V.U.

Kwee, W.S., Veldhuizen, R.W., Golding, R.P., Mullink, H., Stam, J., Donner, R. and Boon, M.E. (1982). Histologic distinction between malignant mesothelioma, benign pleural lesion and carcinoma metastasis. *Virch.Arch. (Pathol.Anat.)*, **397**, 287–299

VIII. ILLUSTRATIONS

Throughout the Atlas several different aspects have been illustrated by microphotographs from the same case.

A list of figures is given below so that readers may co-ordinate the various illustrations from the same case.

Figures 4–6.
Figures 7–9.
Figures 10, 11, 28–31.
Figures 13, 19.
Figures 14, 15.
Figures 17, 18.
Figures 27, 182–189.
Figures 38, 46, 73, 75, 82, 83, 98, 99.
Figures 39, 41, 50, 51, 104, 105.
Figures 40, 47, 48, 52, 95, 174–181.
Figures 42, 43, 74, 76, 100, 101.
Figures 45, 77, 87, 90, 91, 94.
Figures 53, 56–61.
Figures 54, 55, 64, 66, 92.
Figures 62, 63, 67, 71.
Figures 70, 190–195.
Figures 78, 81.
Figures 84, 85, 93.
Figures 86, 146–153.
Figures 88, 89.
Figures 96, 97.
Figures 102, 103.
Figures 106, 107.
Figures 128–145.
Figures 154–173.
Figures 196–203.
Figures 204–209.

All the histopathological illustrations are from slides stained with haematoxylin and eosin, unless otherwise stated.

Gross pathology of diffuse malignant mesothelioma

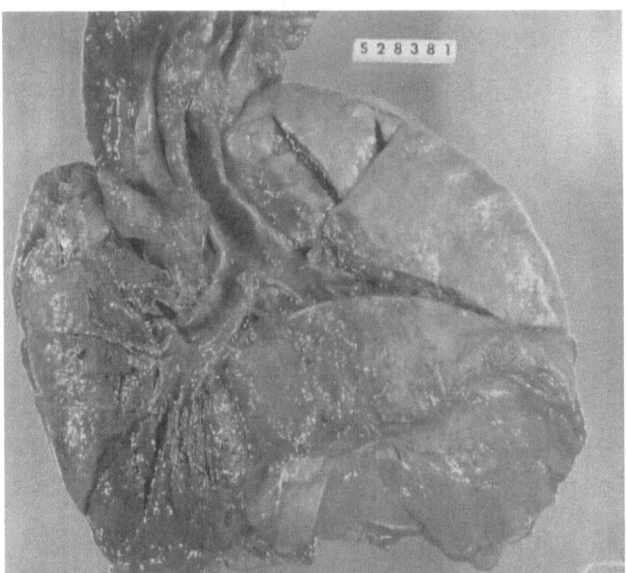

Figure 4 Mesothelioma of right pleura (posterior view) with compression marks of the ribs on the surface. The bronchial tree is dissected in order to exclude the presence of a primary carcinoma of the bronchus

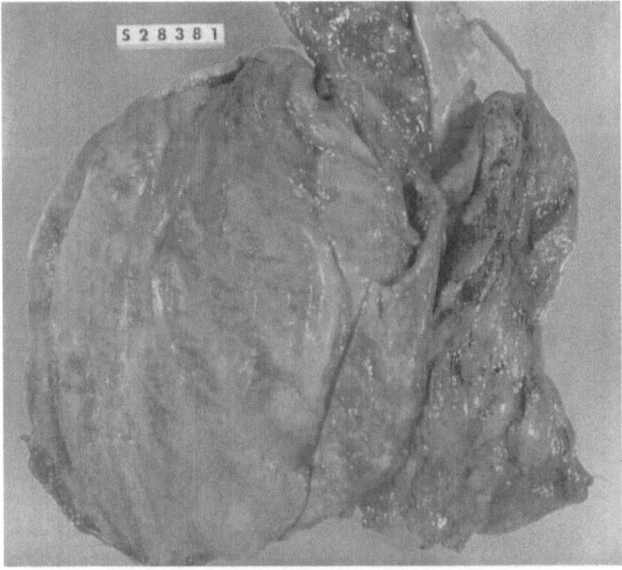

Figure 5 Anterior view of the same specimen

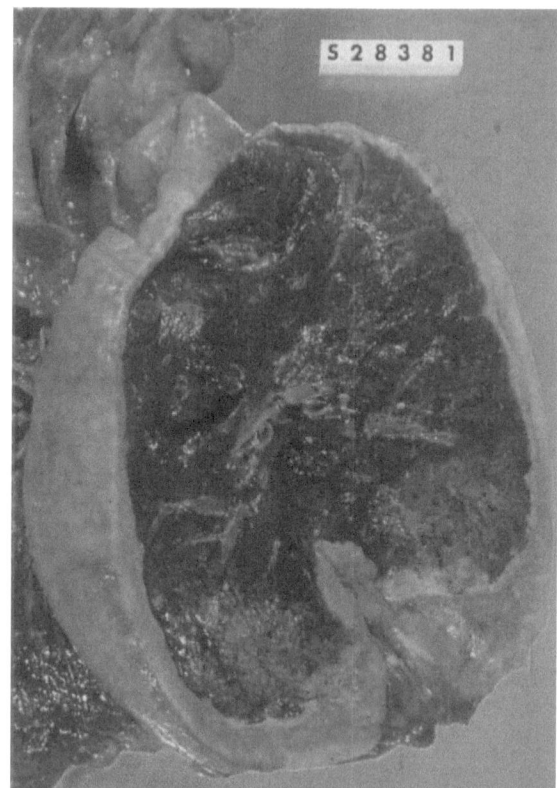

Figure 6   Cut surface of the right lung from the same specimen to demonstrate the total encasement of the lung by pleural mesothelioma. There is linear spread and relatively sharp demarcation between tumour and lung tissue

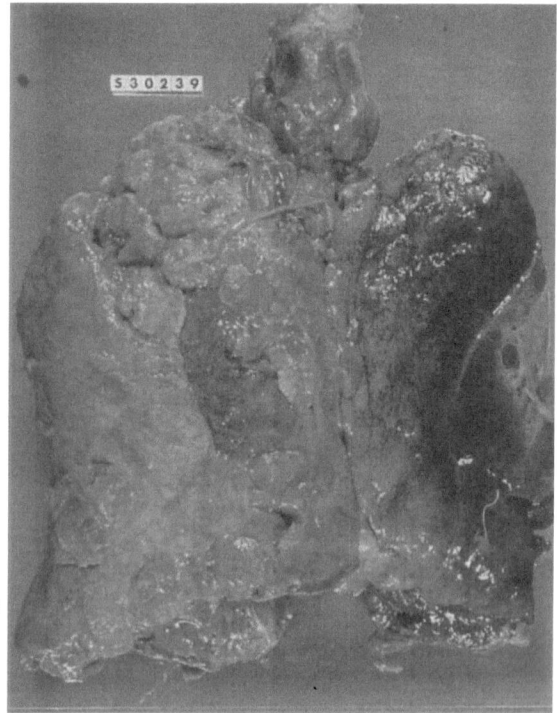

Figure 7   Mesothelioma of the right pleura with focal spread to the base and mid-zone of the left pleura

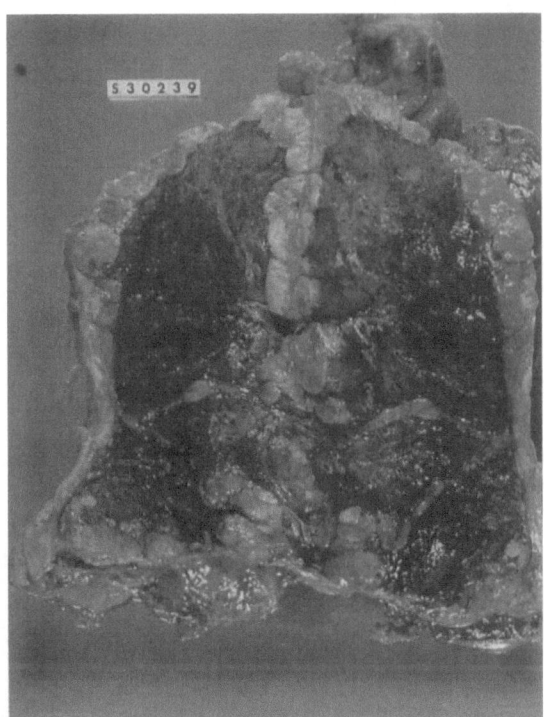

Figure 8 Cut surface of the right lung from the same specimen to demonstrate the nodular pattern of the tumour

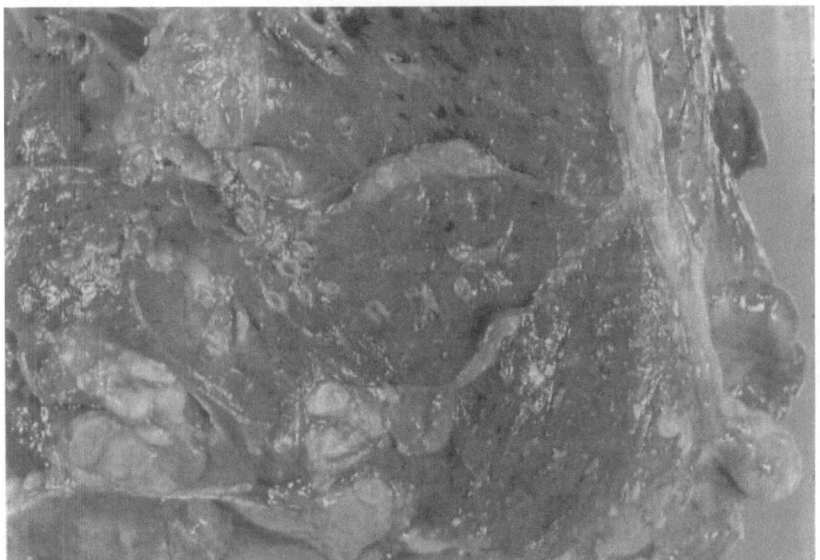

Figure 9 A close-up view of the same case to show in addition the linear spread of tumour along the interlobar fissures

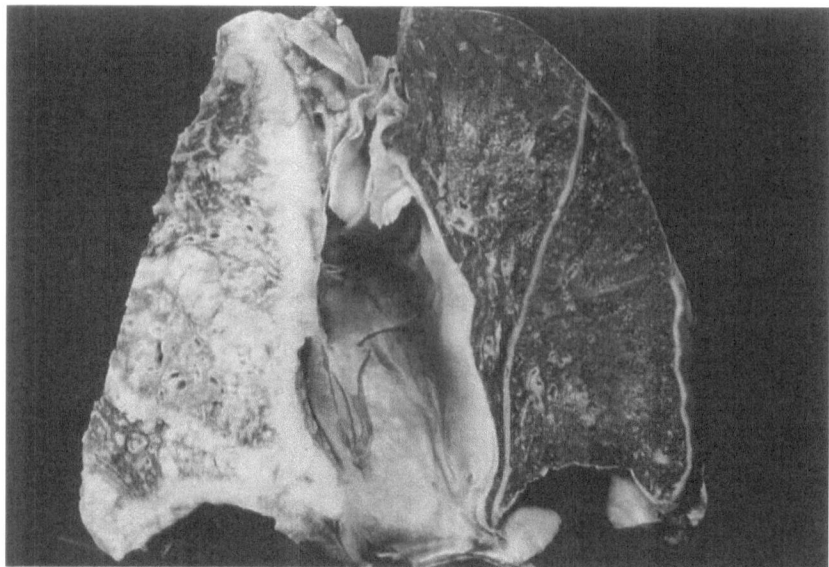

Figure 10   Mesothelioma of the right pleura with spread to the pericardium and left pleura

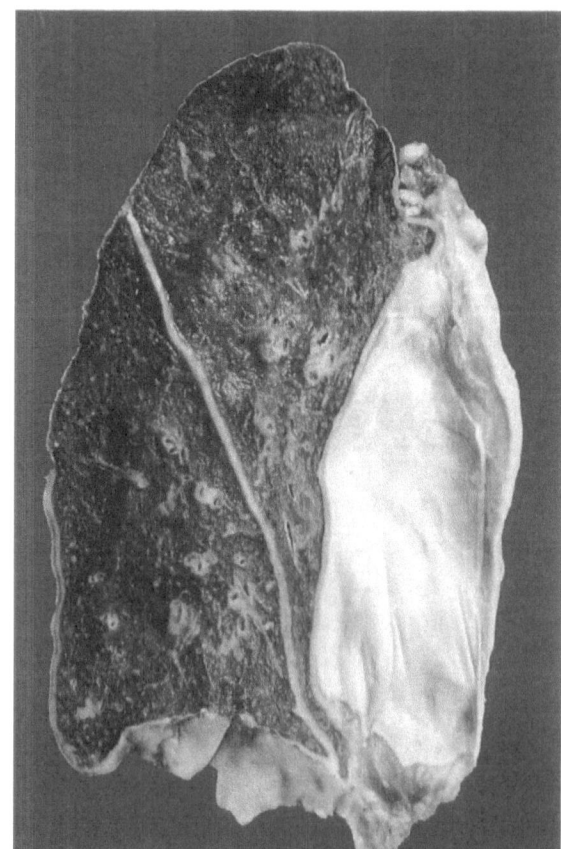

Figure 11   The left lung from the same case to show the thin linear spread of the tumour on the pleural surface and along the interlobar fissure. The white area is the pericardial sac which is also infiltrated by tumour

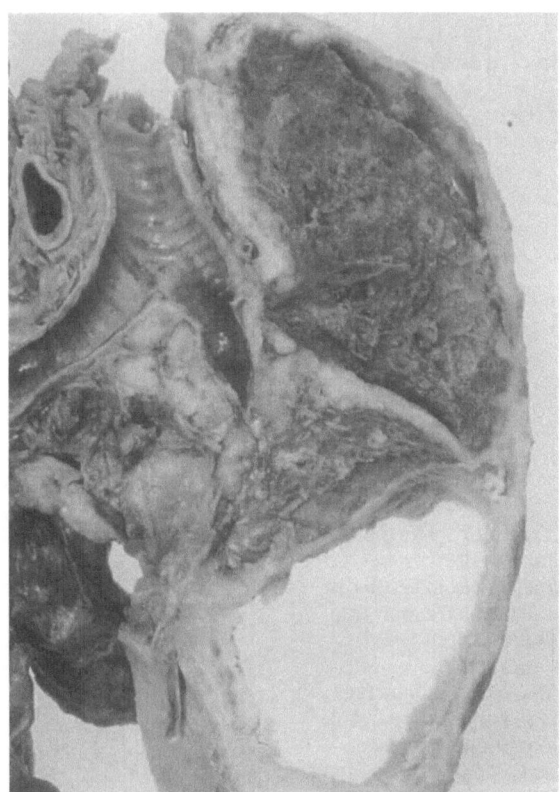

Figure 12   Mesothelioma of the right pleura, showing a large locular space. The effusion has caused compression of the lower lobe of the lung. Note the metastatic deposits of tumour in the mediastinal lymph nodes

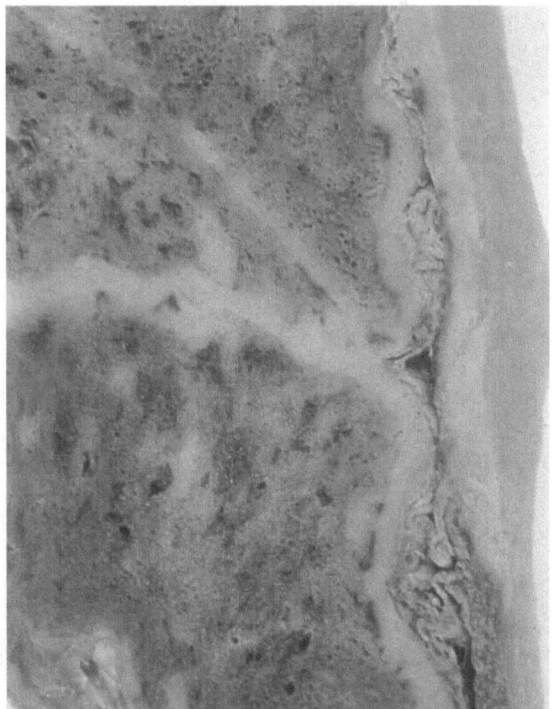

Figure 13   The tumour on the visceral and parietal layers of the pleura is fusing with progressive obliteration of the space. The interlobar space has fused completely. In addition the white foci in the lung parenchyma denote peribronchial lymphatic spread of tumour

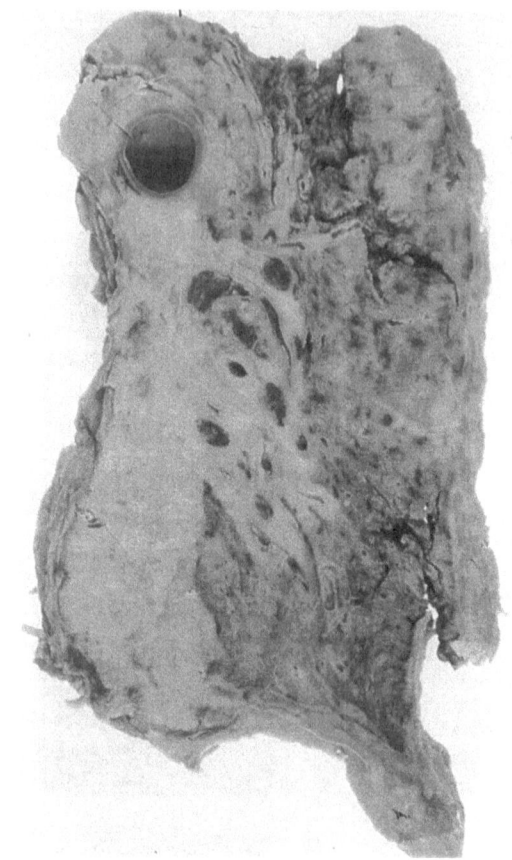

Figure 14   The main mass of the mesothelioma is on the mediastinal aspect and there is spread of tumour to the diaphragmatic surface. The ragged appearance on the outer surface indicates the difficulty of removing the adherent tumour from the chest wall

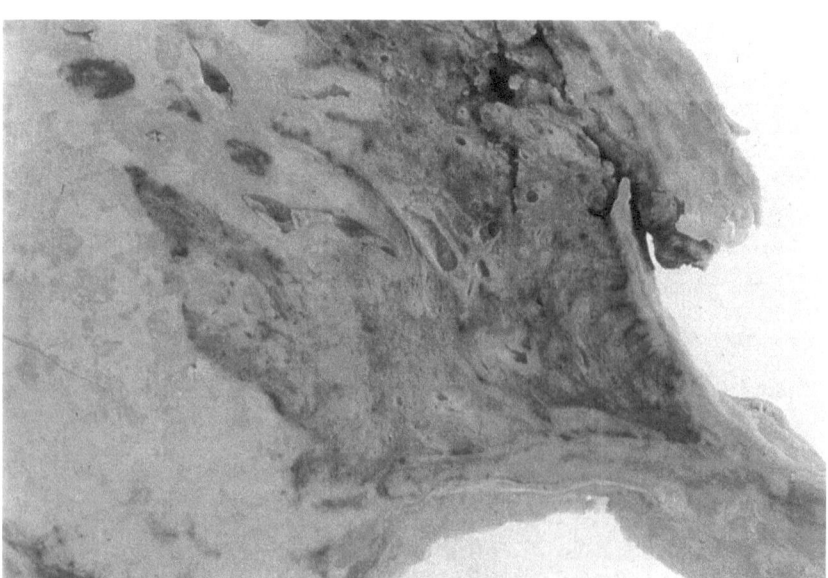

Figure 15   A close-up view of the same case shows the 'macaroni' appearance of the bronchi caused by lymphatic spread of tumour

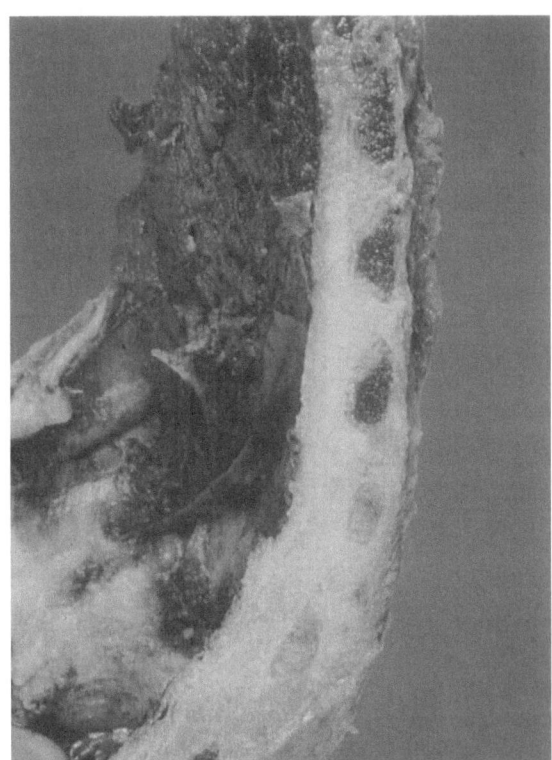

Figure 16   A section through the chest wall shows the firm anchorage of tumour to the intercostal tissues, but leaving most of the ribs intact

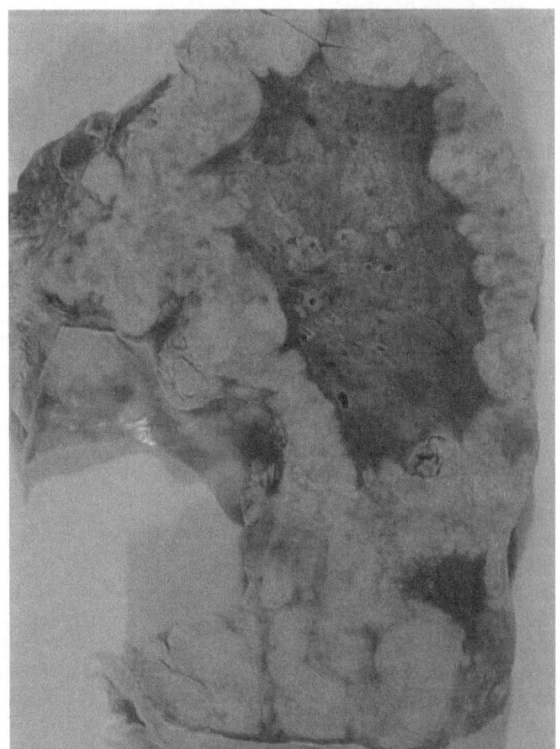

Figure 17   The specimen shows the nodular pattern of a pleural mesothelioma, encasing and compressing the lung (compare with the fresh, unfixed specimen – Figure 8). The parietal layer of pericardium has a smooth surface and is not invaded by tumour

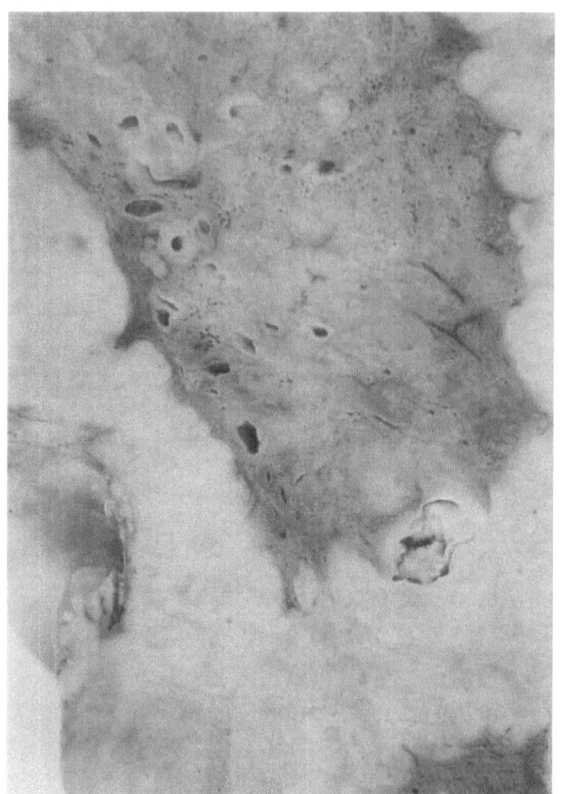

Figure 18   A close-up view of the same case demonstrating a small yellow area of necrosis

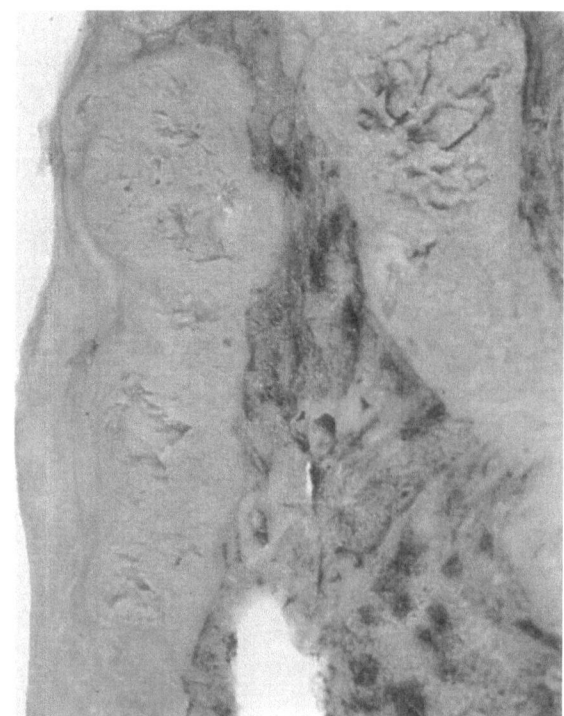

Figure 19   The necrotic appearance along the pleural plane could be due to organization of an old haemorrhagic effusion, or to necrosis of the tumour itself. The latter possibility is very rare in mesotheliomas (same case as in Figure 13)

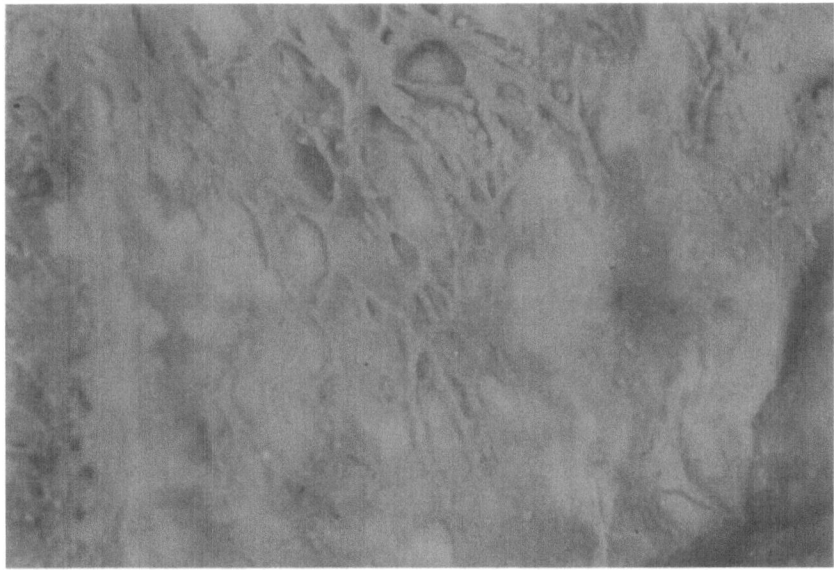

Figure 20 A view of the visceral pleura showing the roughened, web-like surface of a mesothelioma, as it would be seen on thoracoscopy

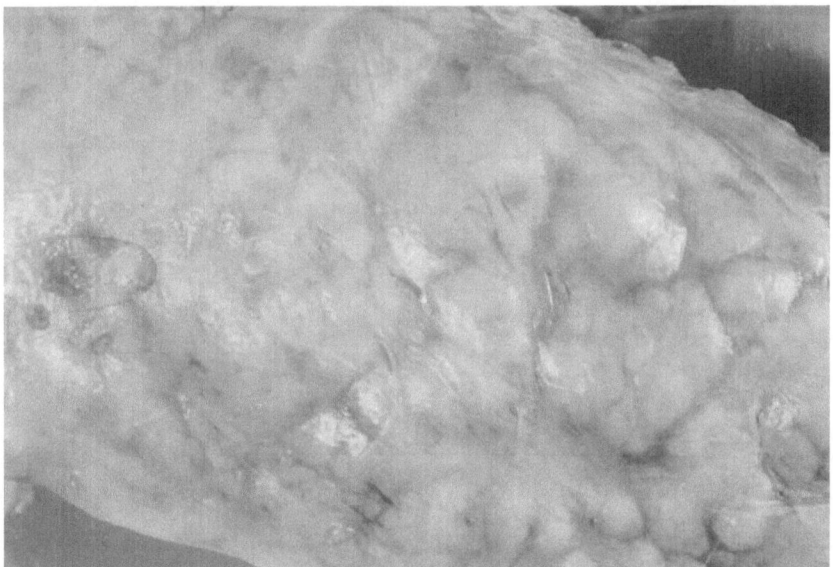

Figure 21 A view of the visceral pleura showing the surface of a nodular, but smooth mesothelioma as it would be seen on thoracoscopy

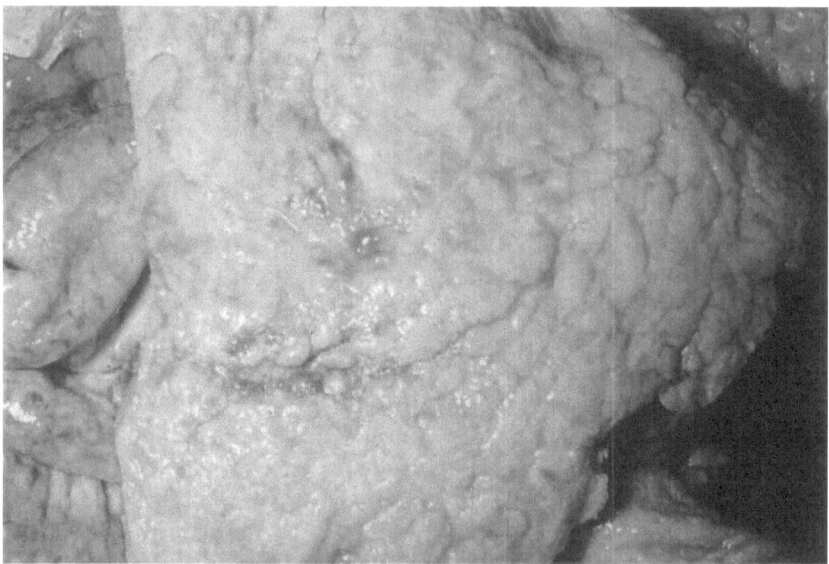

Figure 22 Mesothelioma of the peritoneum. The diffuse infiltration of omental tissue is indistinguishable from metastatic carcinoma

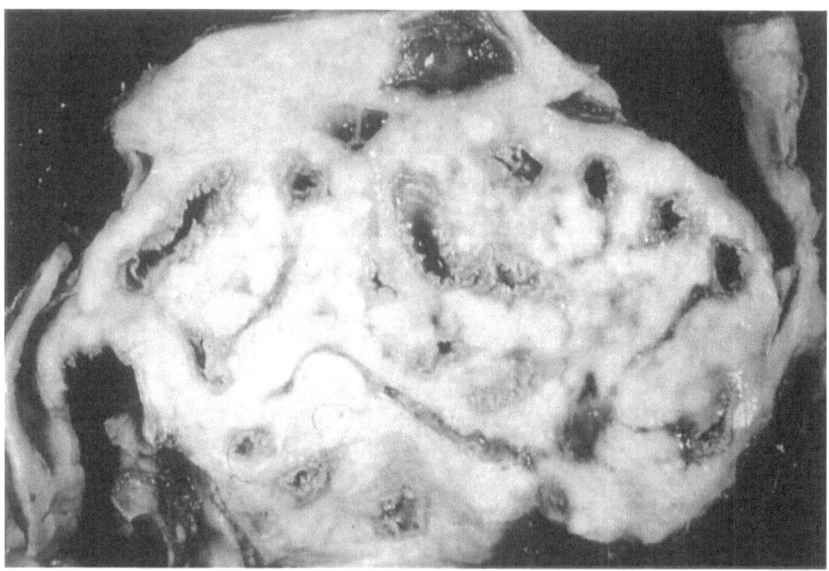

Figure 23 Mesothelioma of the peritoneum. A transverse section through the small and large intestines which are fused together by a thick white tumour mass. This is confined to the serosal surface, leaving the inner layers of the intestinal wall intact

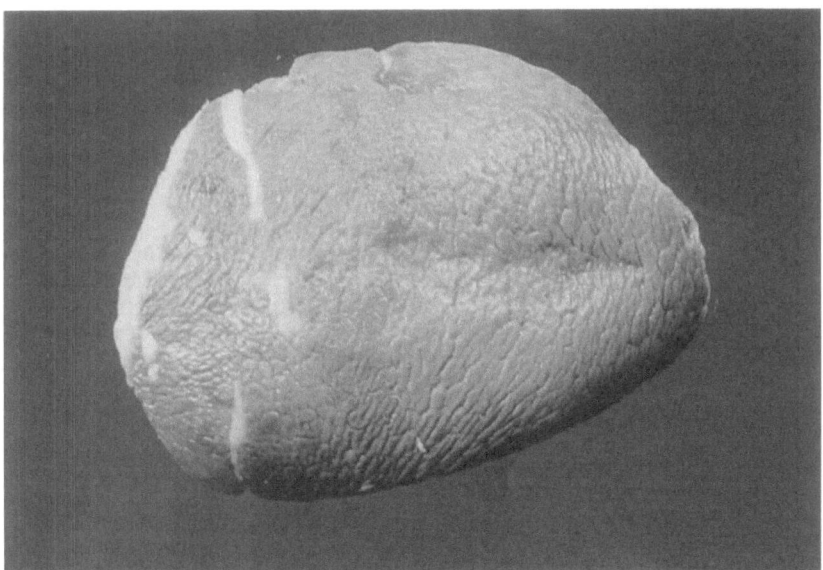

Figure 24   A thin sheet of mesothelioma on the serosal surface of the spleen

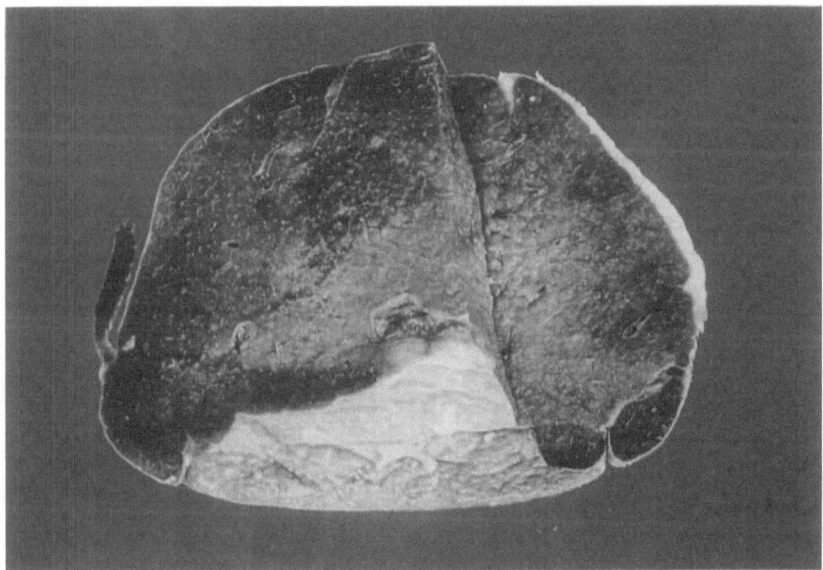

Figure 25   The cut surface of the same specimen

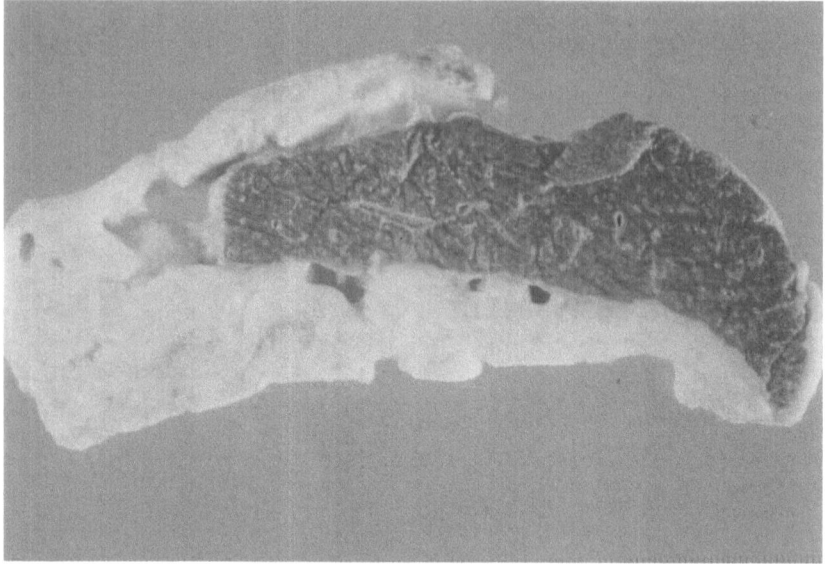

Figure 26   A thick layer of peritoneal mesothelioma on the serosal surface of the spleen. There is no invasion of the parenchyma

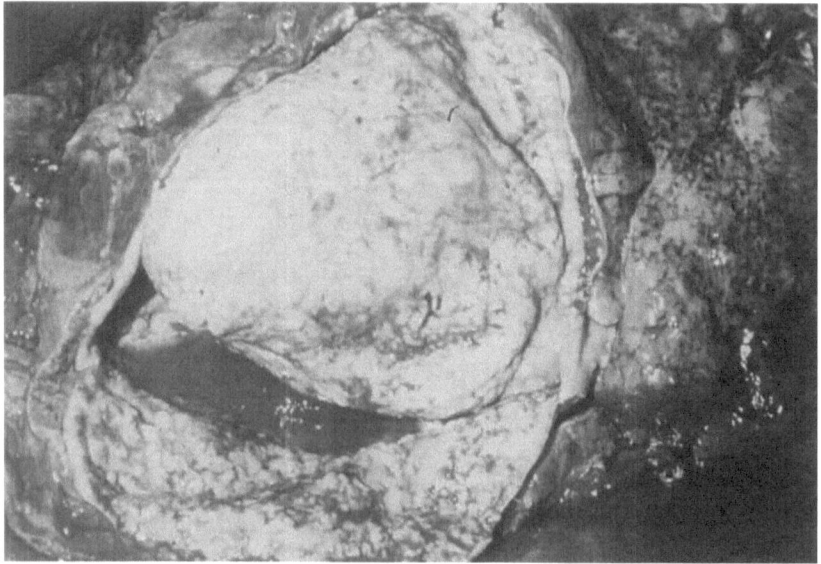

Figure 27   Mesothelioma of the pericardium affecting both visceral and parietal layers selectively. Normal pleura is seen on both sides

Gross pathology – Metastases

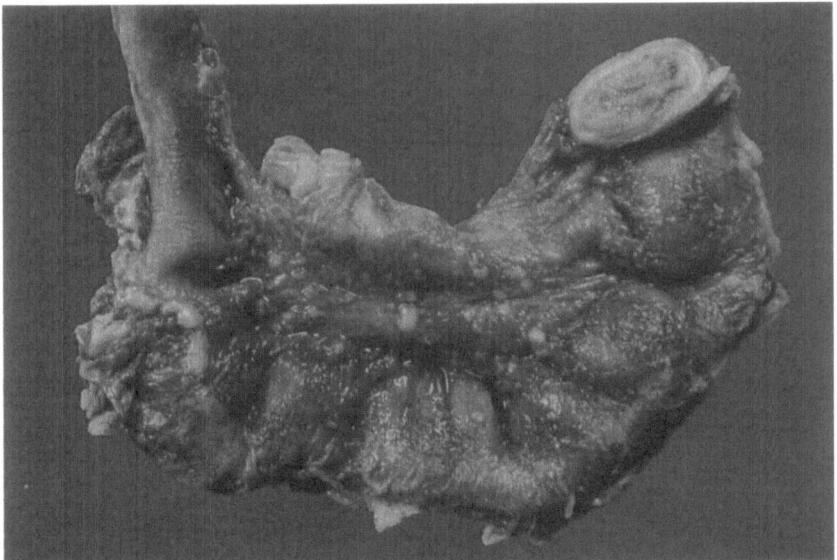

Figure 28 Transcoelomic metastatic spread on the serosal surface of the small intestine and mesentery secondary to a mesothelioma of the pleura (same case as Figure 10)

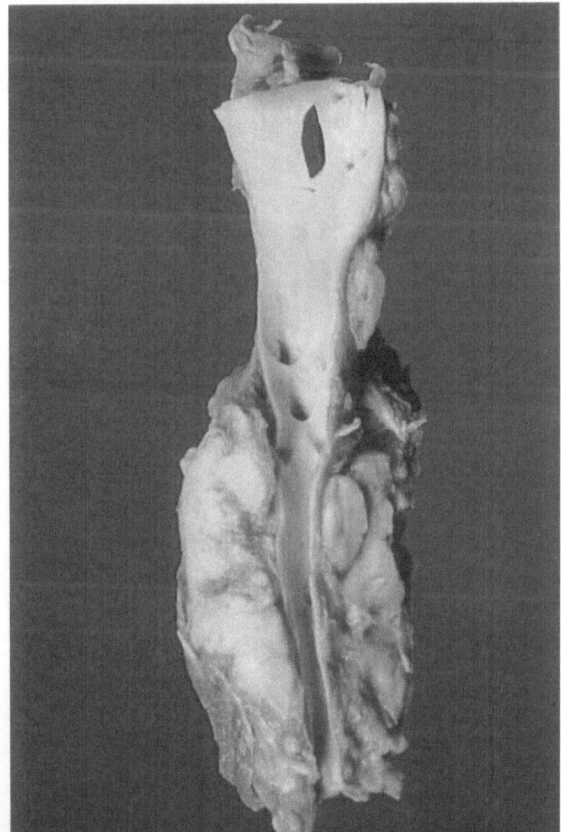

Figure 29 Metastatic spread in the para-aortic lymph nodes secondary to a mesothelioma of the pleura (same case as Figure 10)

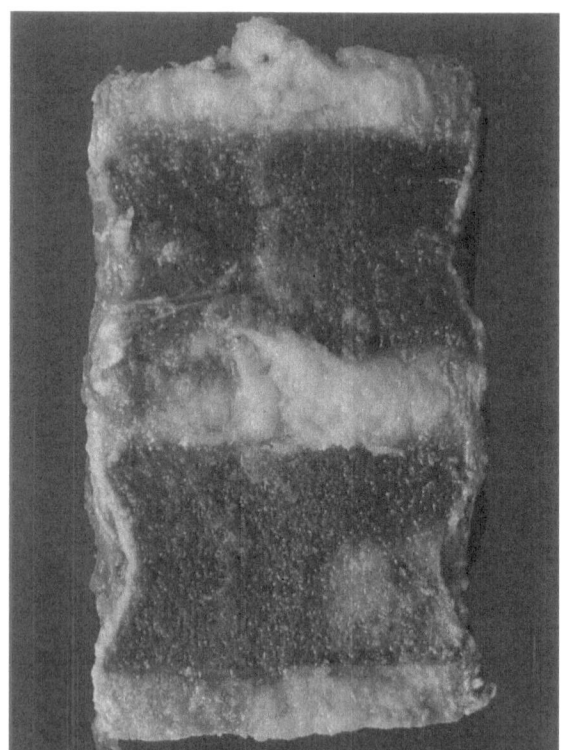

Figure 30   Blood-borne spread to bone has been derived from a primary mesothelioma of the pleura (same case as Figure 10)

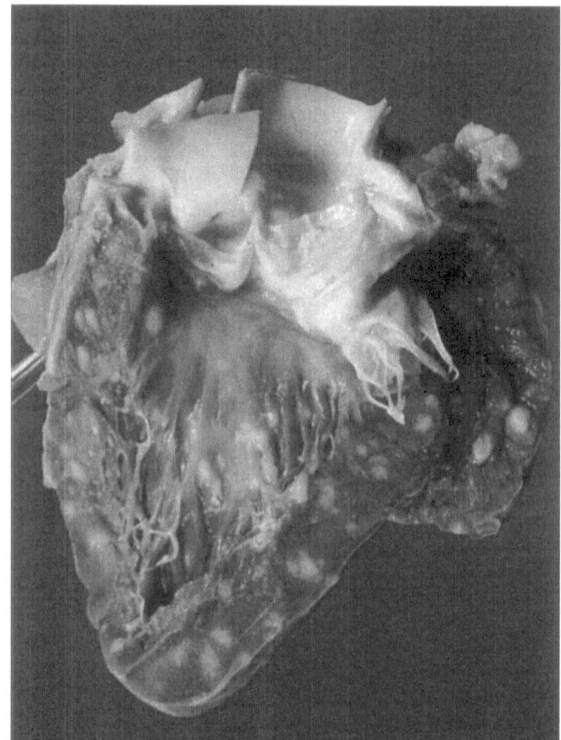

Figure 31   Blood-borne spread to the myocardium and subserosal tissue has been derived from a primary mesothelioma of the pleura (same case as Figure 10)

Gross pathology – Differential diagnosis

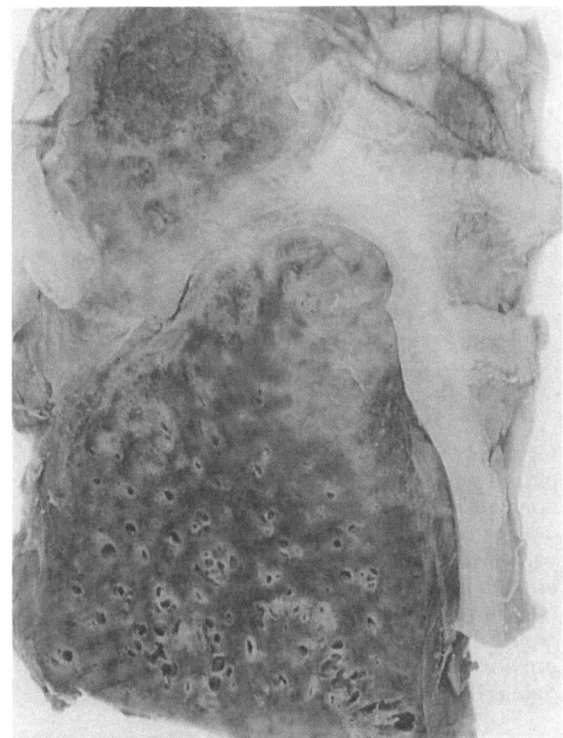

Figure 32   The thick reactive fibrosis of the pleura closely resembles the gross appearance of a mesothelioma. There is however a very sharp demarcation between the pleura and lung parenchyma. The underlying lung tissue shows asbestosis

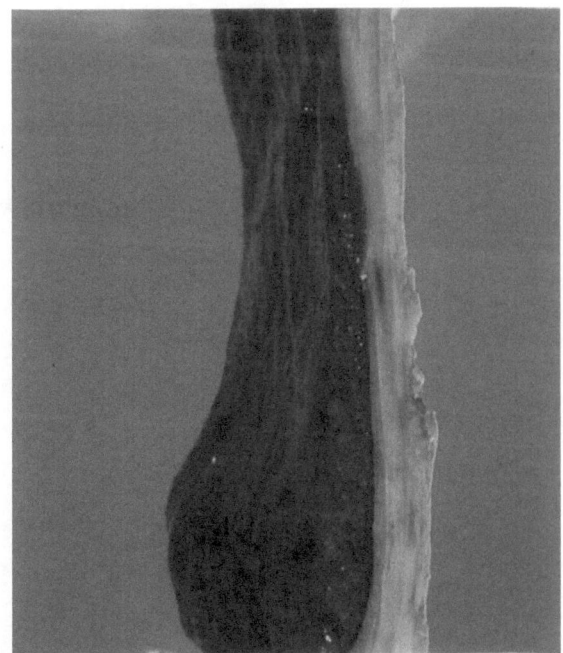

Figure 33   Fresh specimen of the visceral pleura showing a hyaline appearance and sharp demarcation of the reactive fibrous thickening

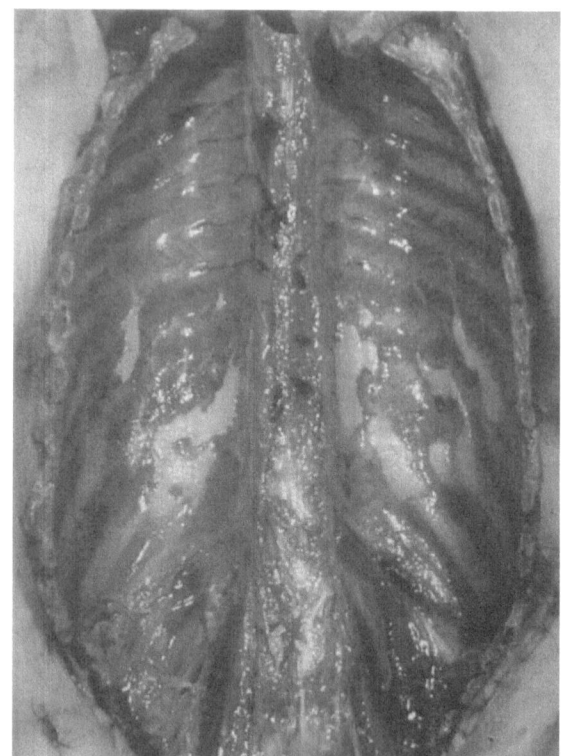

Figure 34 Yellow pleural plaques are symmetrically distributed on the parietal pleura in the lower thorax, mainly following the line of the ribs (slide kindly provided by Dr P.G. Smith)

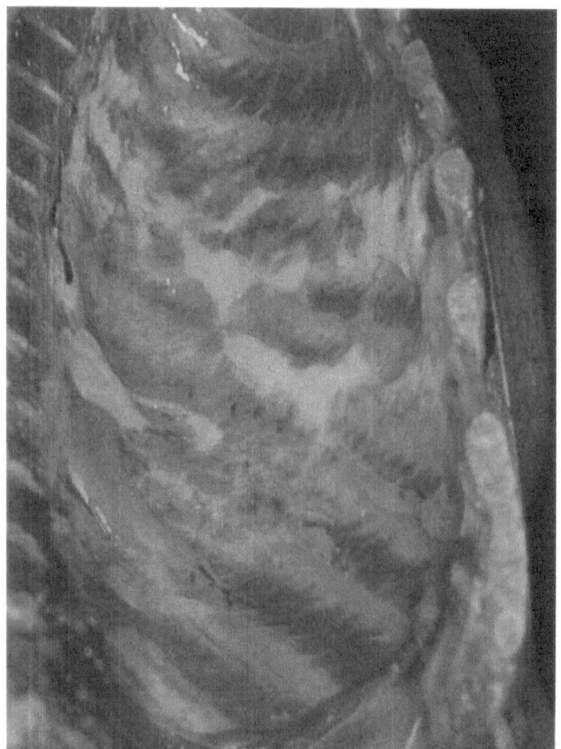

Figure 35 White pleural plaques are situated in the left mid-thoracic cavity, less sharply demarcated than those in Figure 34 (slide kindly provided by Dr P.G. Smith)

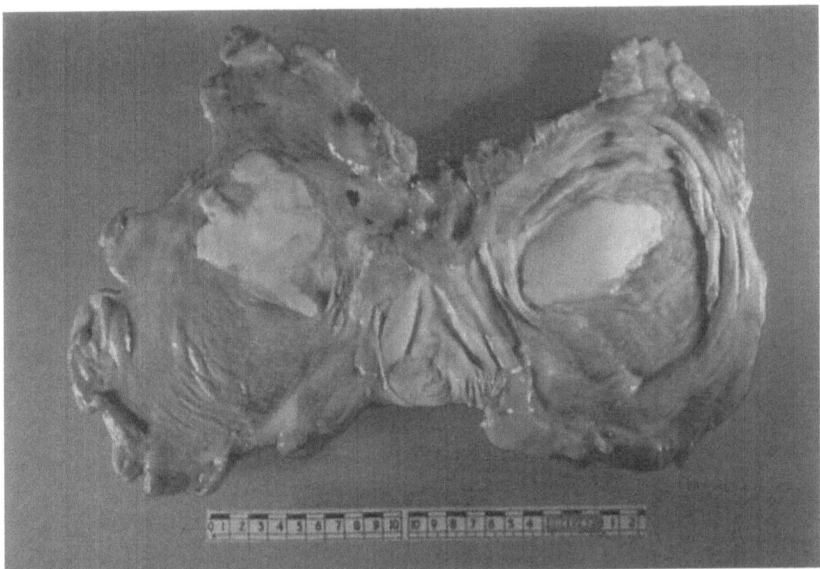

Figure 36 Specimen of the diaphragm shows the distribution of flat pleural plaques on the central tendon

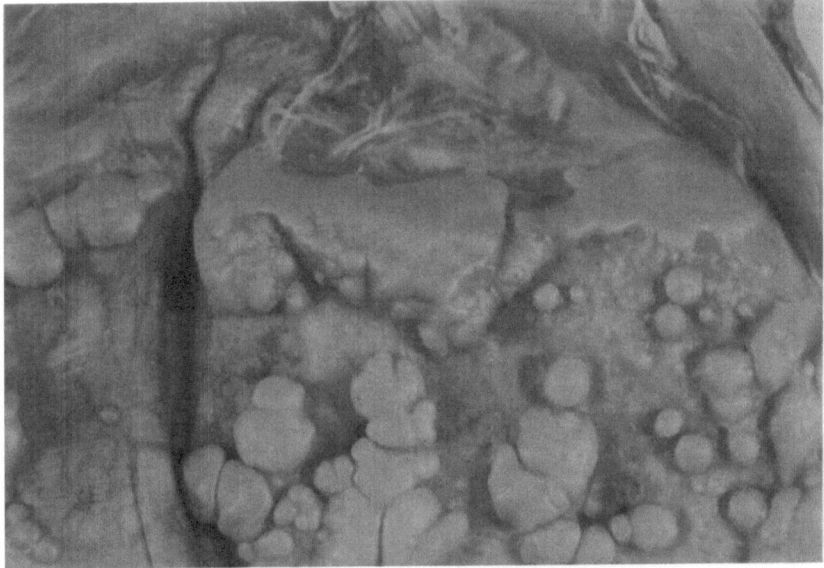

Figure 37 A close-up view of flat and nodular pleural plaques situated on the central tendon of the diaphragm

Histopathology of diffuse malignant mesothelioma

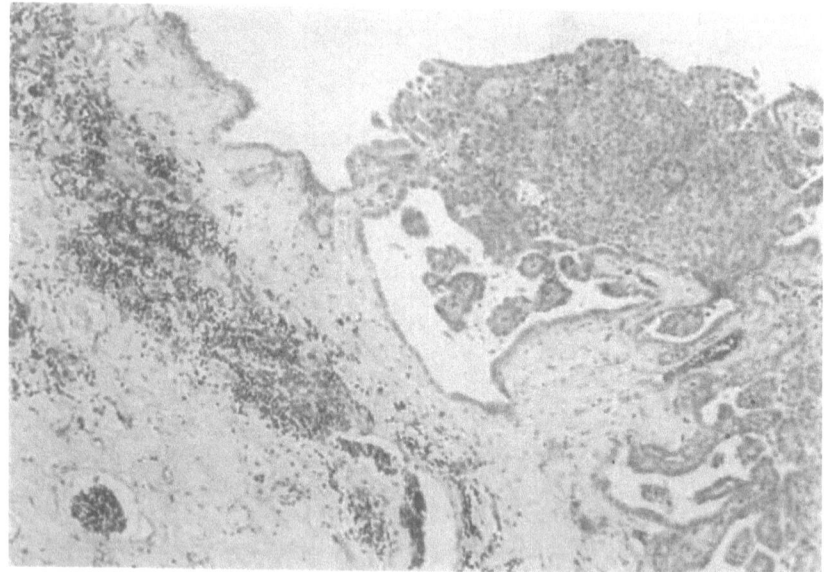

Figure 38   Low power view of a typical mesothelioma of the pleura with an exophytic papillary growth (× 110)

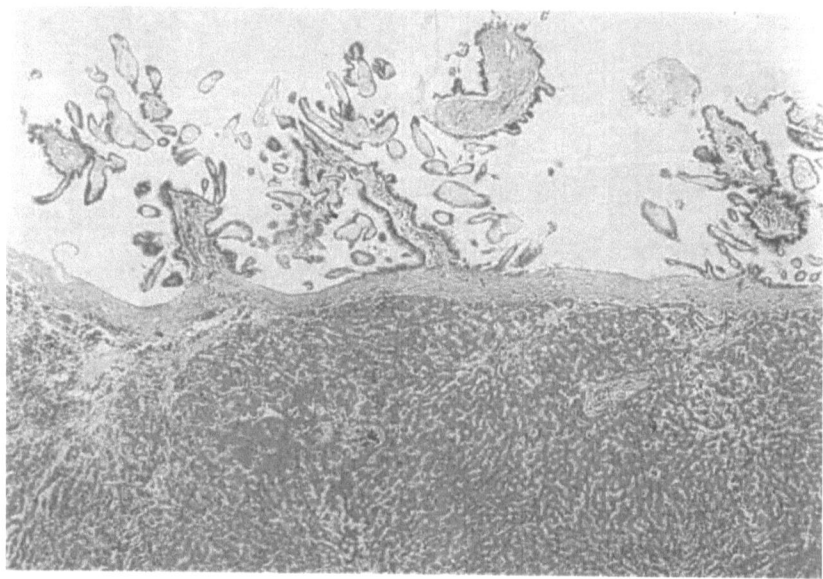

Figure 39   Low power view of a peritoneal mesothelioma with an exophytic papillary growth on the surface of the liver (× 45)

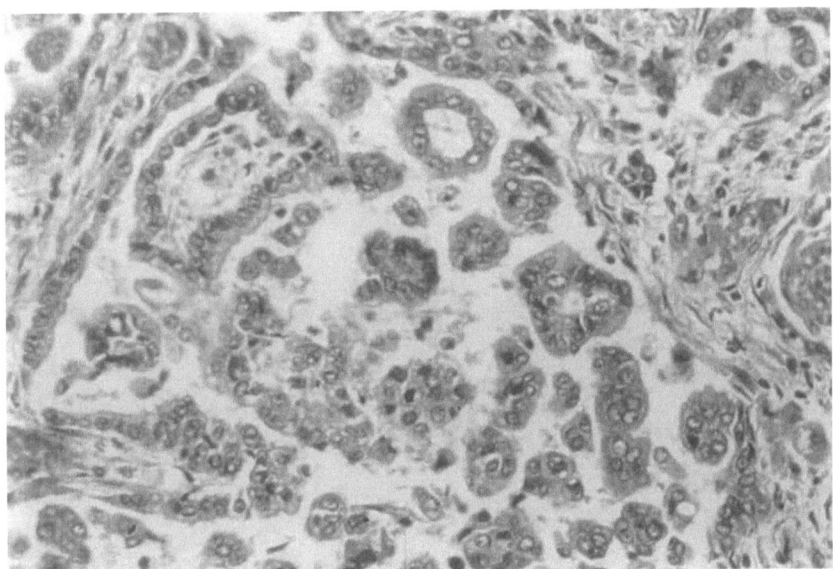

Figure 40   Epithelial type, papillary pattern (× 275)

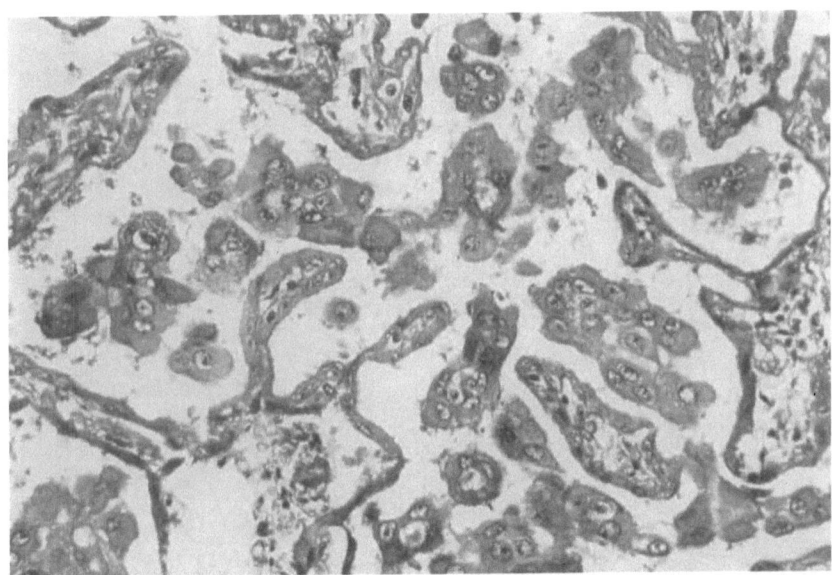

Figure 41   Epithelial type, papillary pattern (× 275)

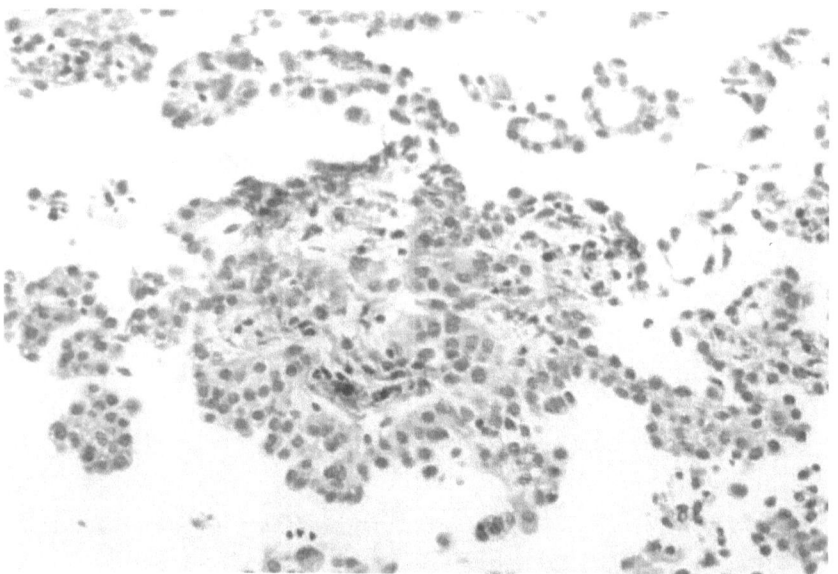

Figure 42   Epithelial type, papillary pattern; low power view (× 275)

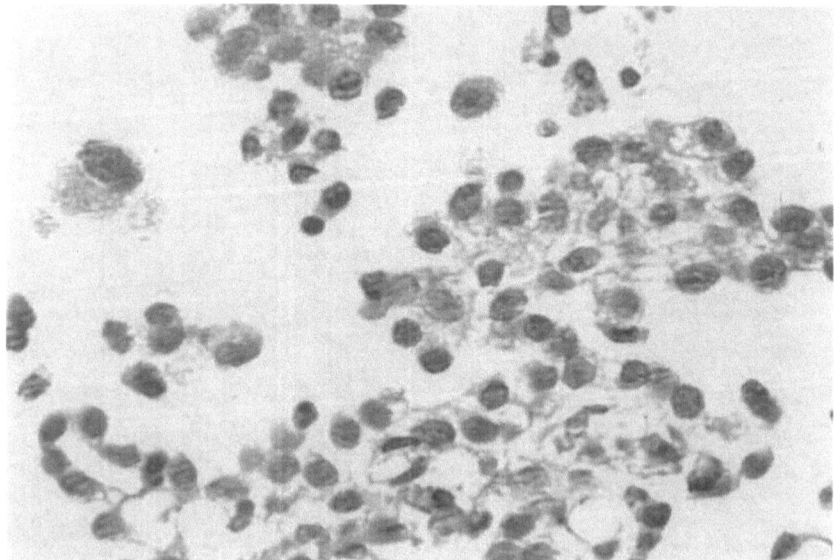

Figure 43   Epithelial type, papillary pattern; high power view, showing the uniform cellular appearance (× 730)

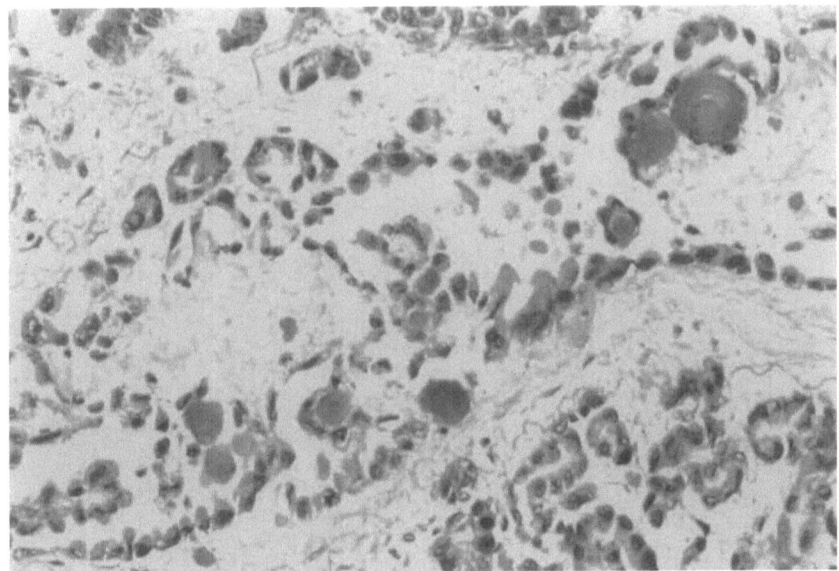

Figure 44 Epithelial type, papillary pattern, showing psammoma bodies (× 275)

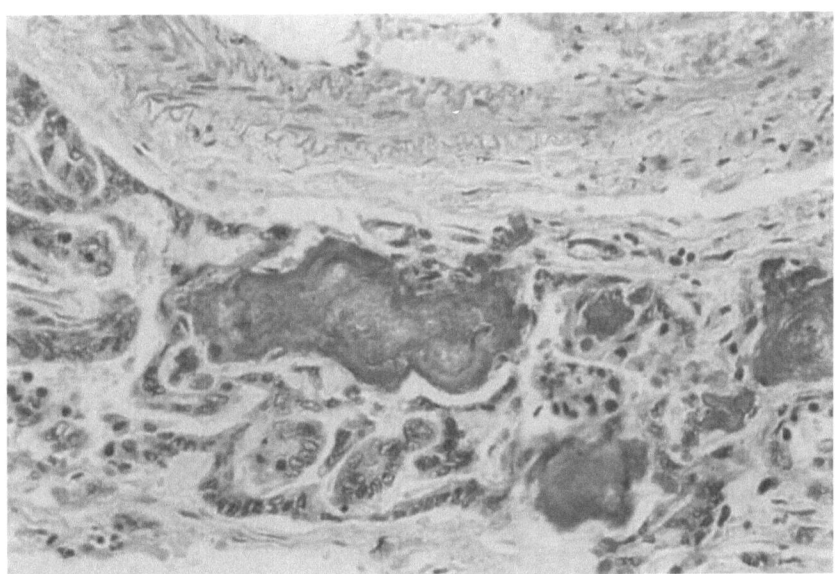

Figure 45 Epithelial type, papillary pattern, showing irregular calcified structures (× 275)

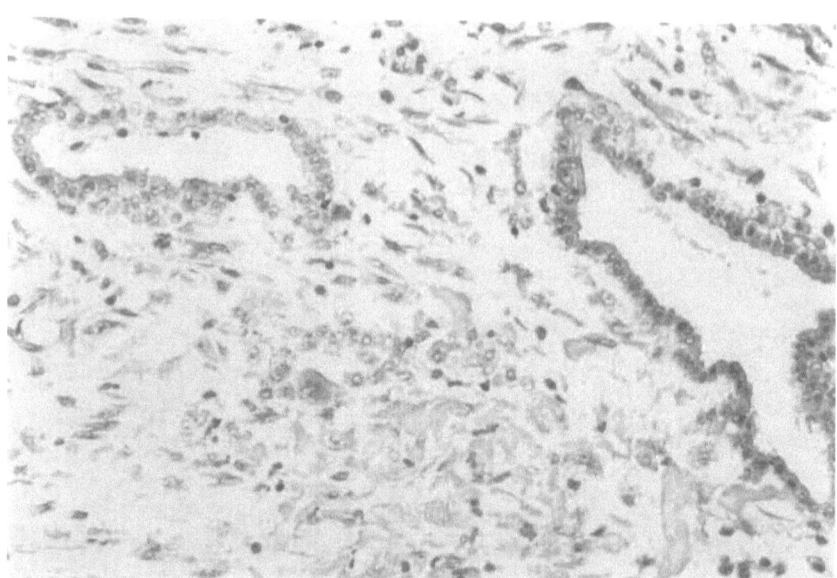

Figure 46   Epithelial type, mainly tubular pattern (× 275)

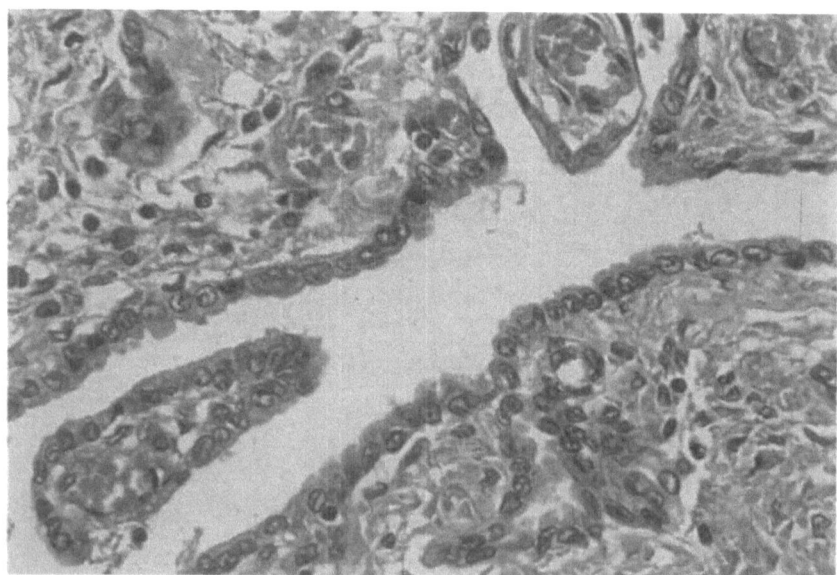

Figure 47   Epithelial type, tubular pattern; higher magnification, showing a single layer of uniform cuboidal cells (× 430)

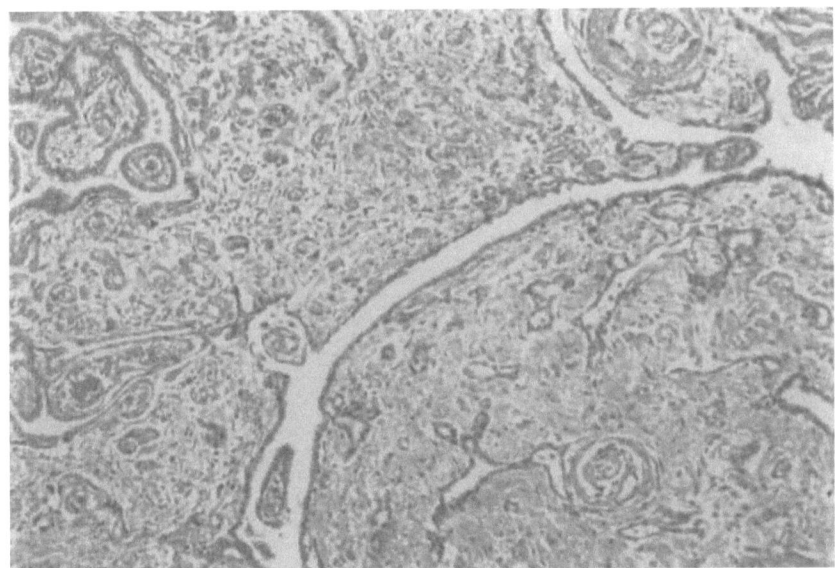

Figure 48 Epithelial type, tubulo-papillary pattern. The clefts are lined by flattened epithelial type cells (× 110)

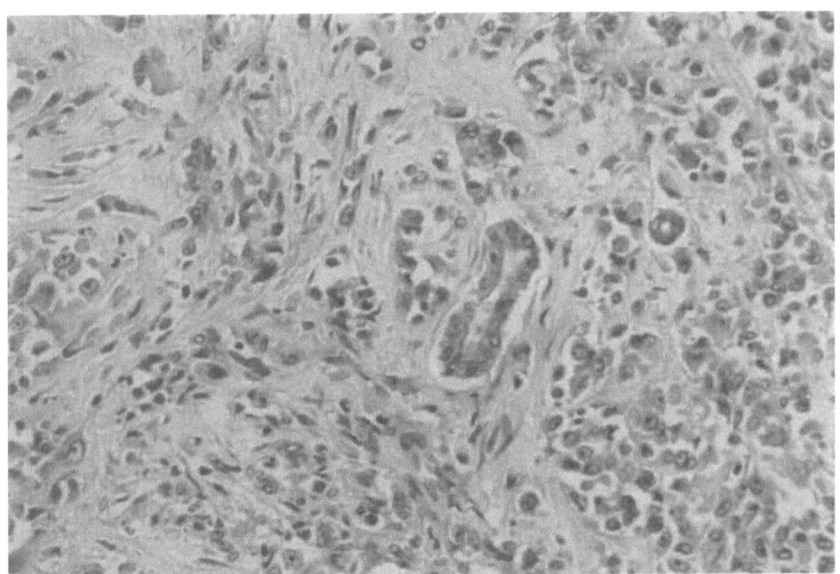

Figure 49 Epithelial type, tubular pattern, with varying degrees of differentiation (× 275)

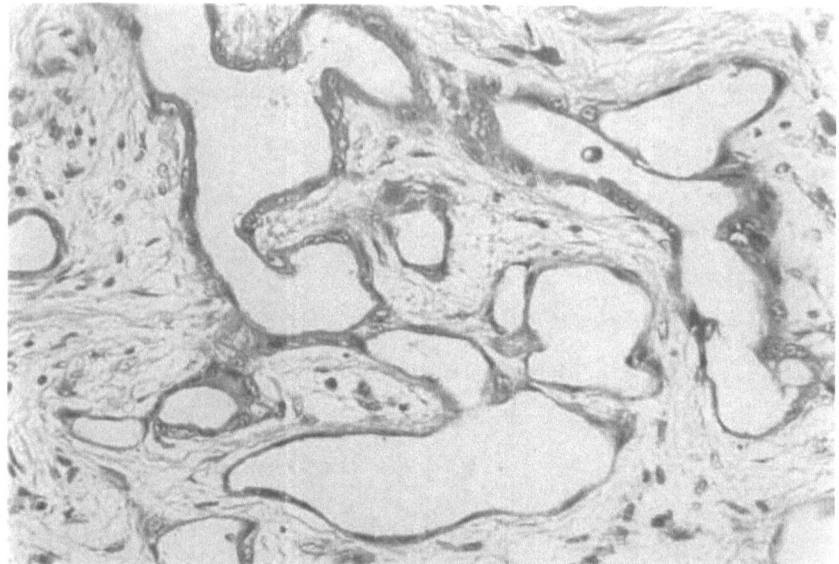

Figure 50 Epithelial type, tubular pattern with a microcystic appearance. The lining cells vary from cuboidal to flattened (× 275)

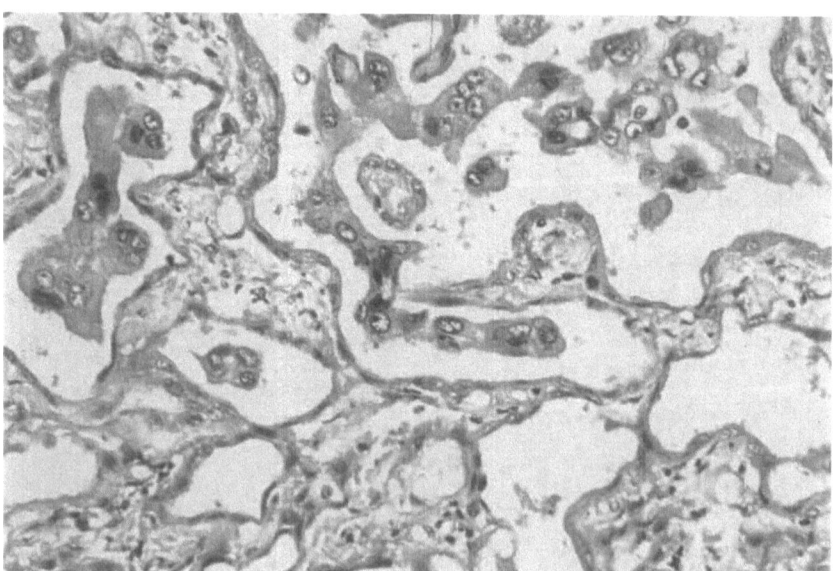

Figure 51 Part of the same tumour as in Figure 50, but in addition there is a papillary component in which the cells show pronounced pleomorphism (× 275)

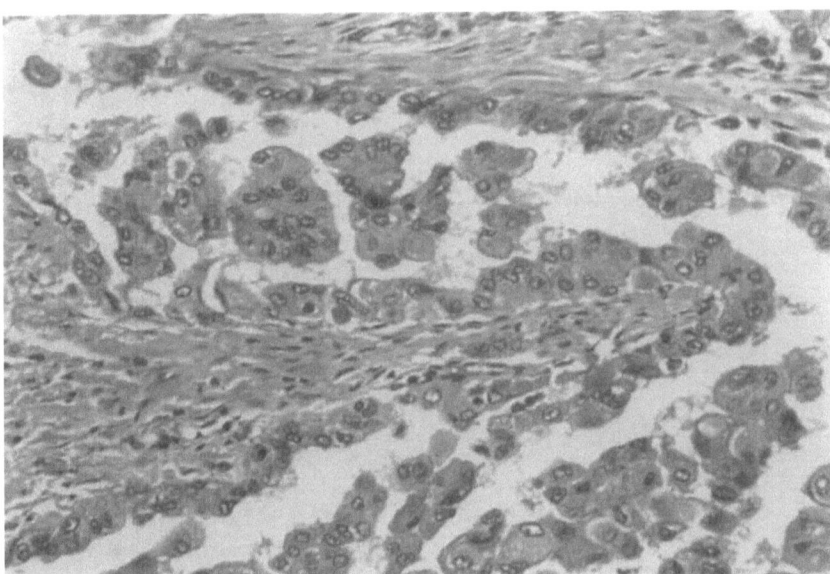

Figure 52 Epithelial type, tubulo-papillary pattern. Clusters of cells appear to have separated from the lining cell layer. The stroma has a dense appearance (× 275)

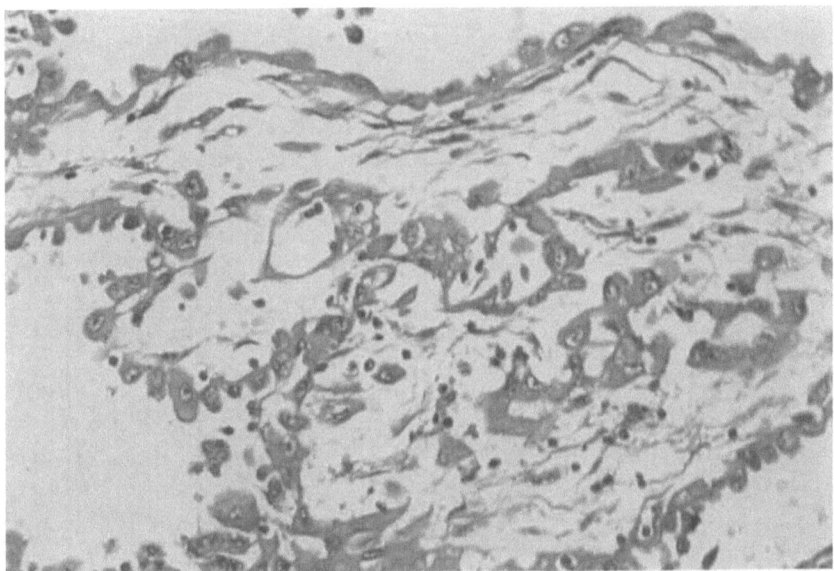

Figure 53 Epithelial type, tubulo-papillary pattern. The nuclei of some of the surface cells bulge into the spaces. In contrast to Figure 52, the connective tissue has a loose arrangement (× 275)

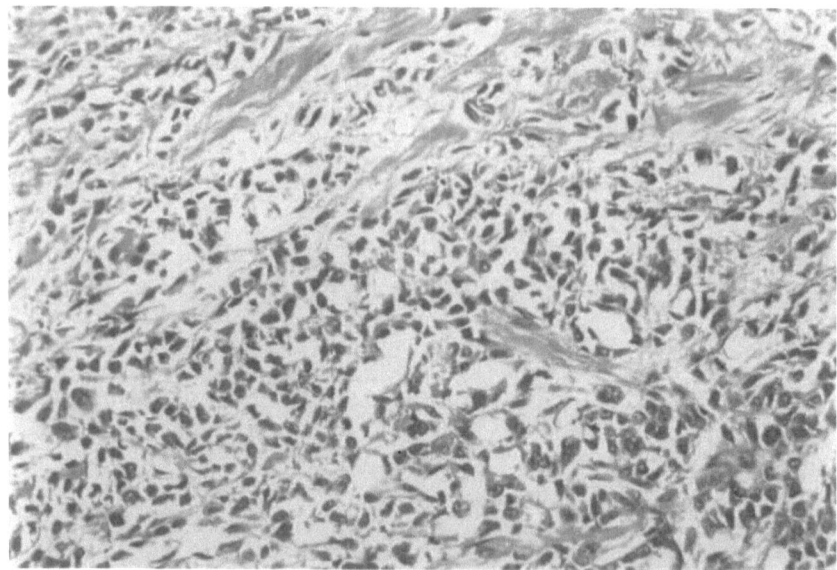

Figure 54   Epithelial type, small cell variety, found in an otherwise typical meso-thelioma. Some larger cells are also seen in the bottom right hand corner (× 275)

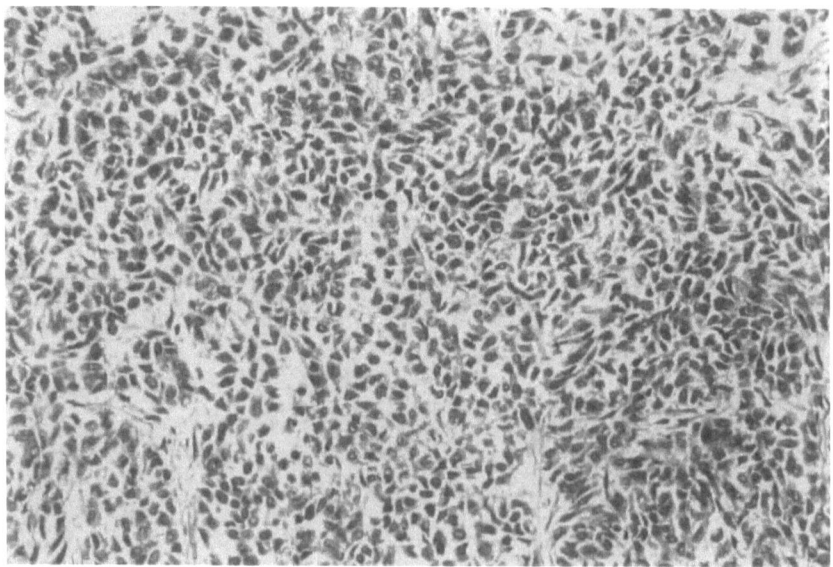

Figure 55   A cellular-rich area from the same case as in Figure 54, showing uniform small cells which mimic a small cell anaplastic carcinoma (× 275)

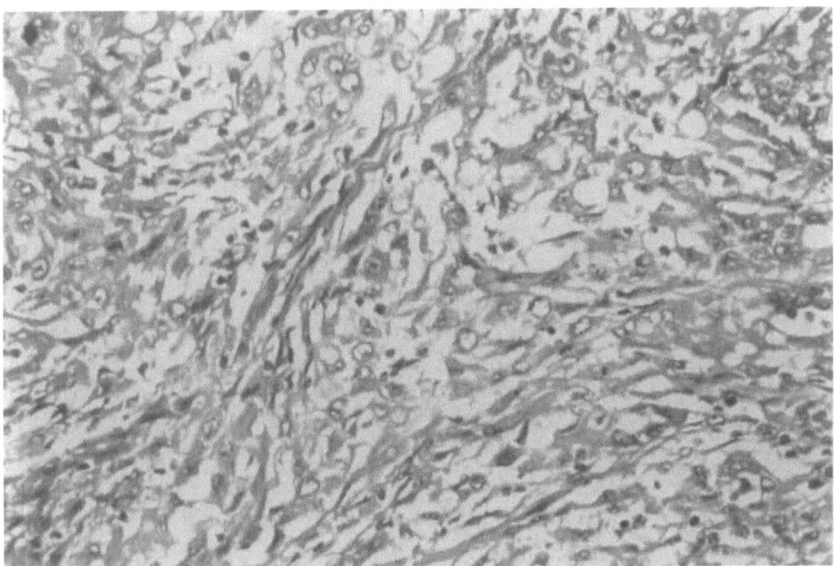

Figure 56 A mainly epithelial type with an undifferentiated appearance. A connective tissue component is also present (× 275)

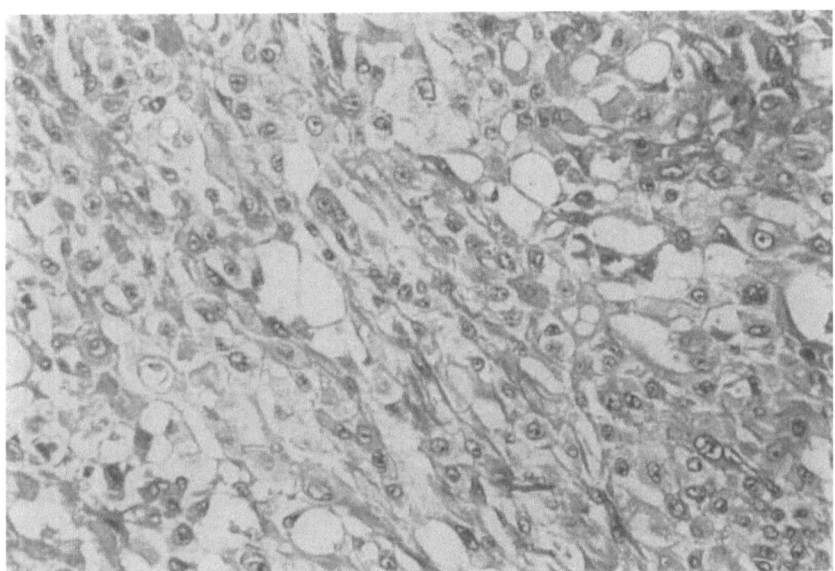

Figure 57 Another view from the same case as in Figure 56, which shows more clearly the predominance of the epithelial element (× 275)

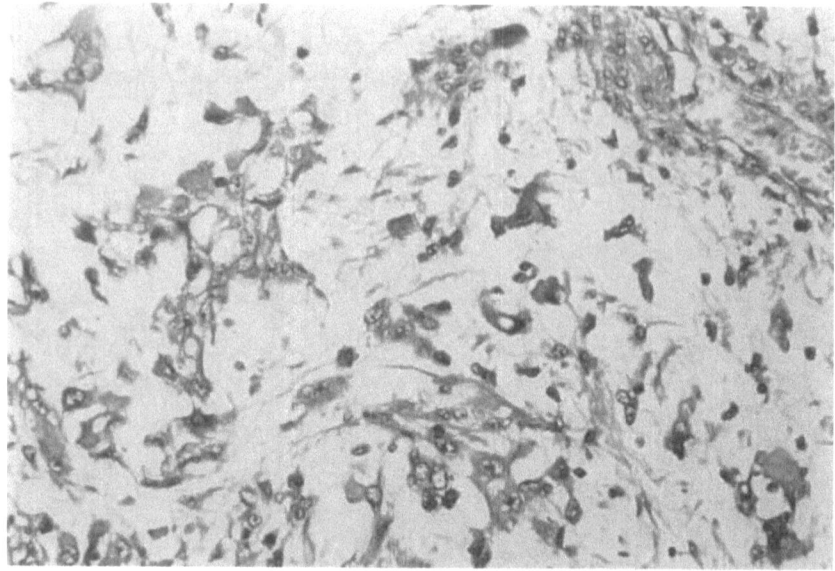

Figure 58 Another view from the same case as in Figure 56, which shows the separation of epithelial cells within a loose connective tissue stroma (× 275)

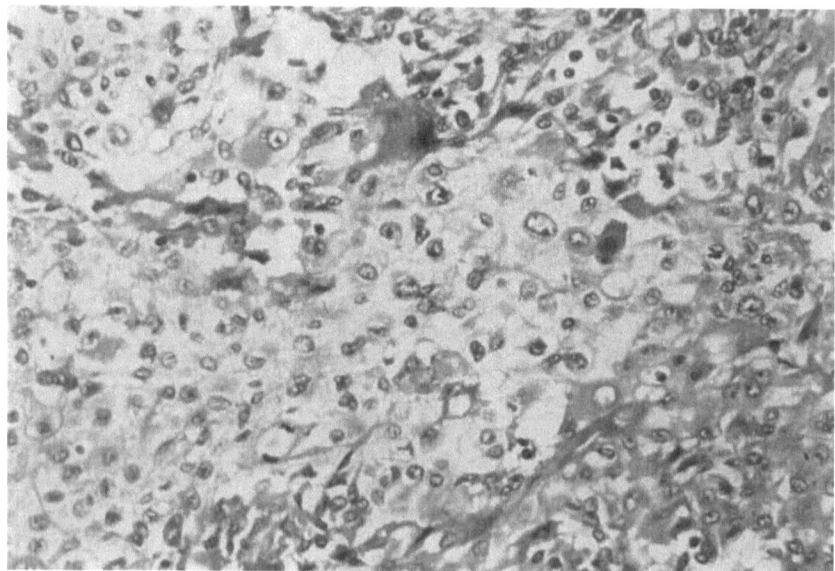

Figure 59 Another view from the same case as in Figure 56 which shows a solid sheet of large epithelial cells. Compare with the small cells of Figure 55 (× 275)

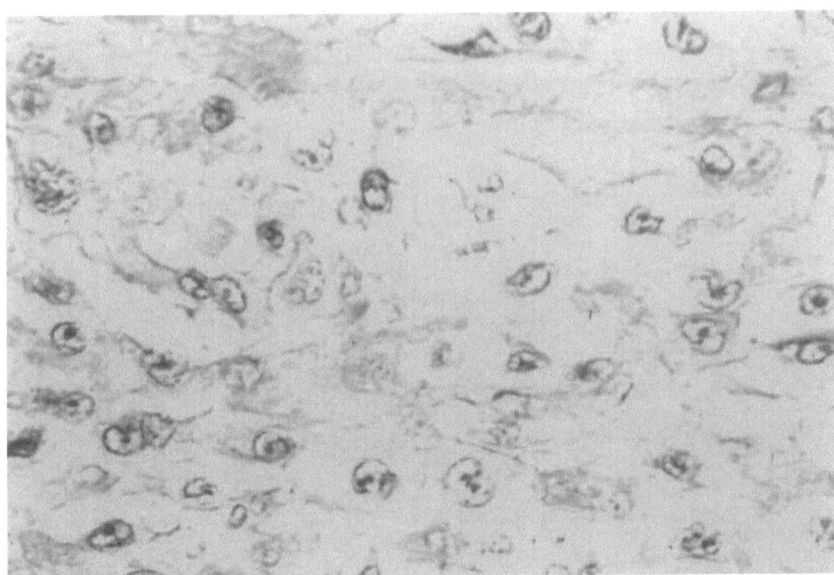

Figure 60 A high power view of the same case as in Figure 56 which shows the large cell variety of epithelial cells. The abundant cytoplasm is weakly acidophilic; the nuclear membrane is well defined; the nuclei are large and vesicular, with prominent nucleoli (× 730)

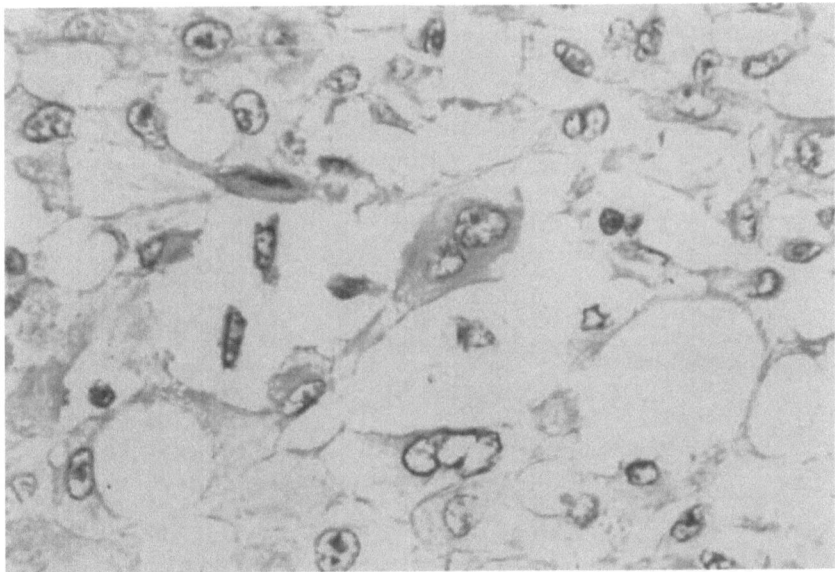

Figure 61 Same case and magnification as in Figure 60 showing vacuoles in the cytoplasm. In the centre there is a large multinucleate cell. Some small shrunken cells are also seen (× 730)

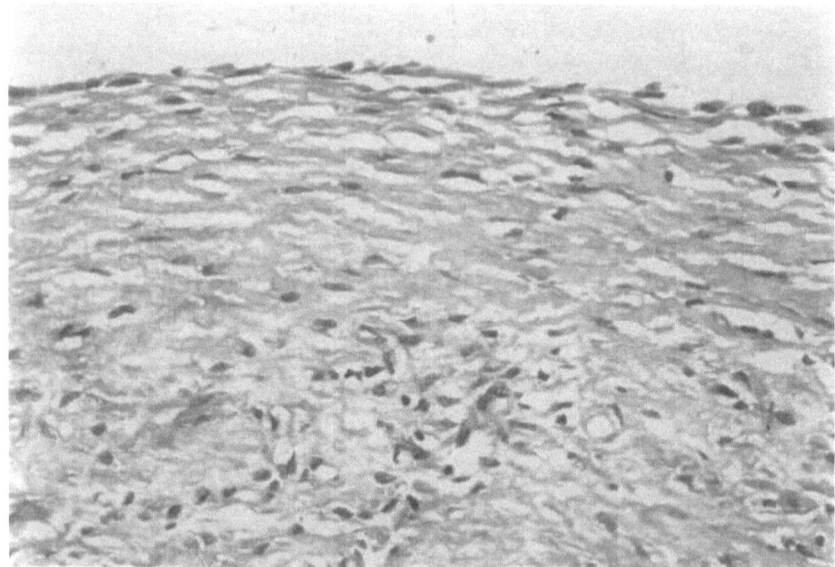

Figure 62 Connective tissue type with poor cellularity especially in the superficial half which mimics a pleural plaque (× 275)

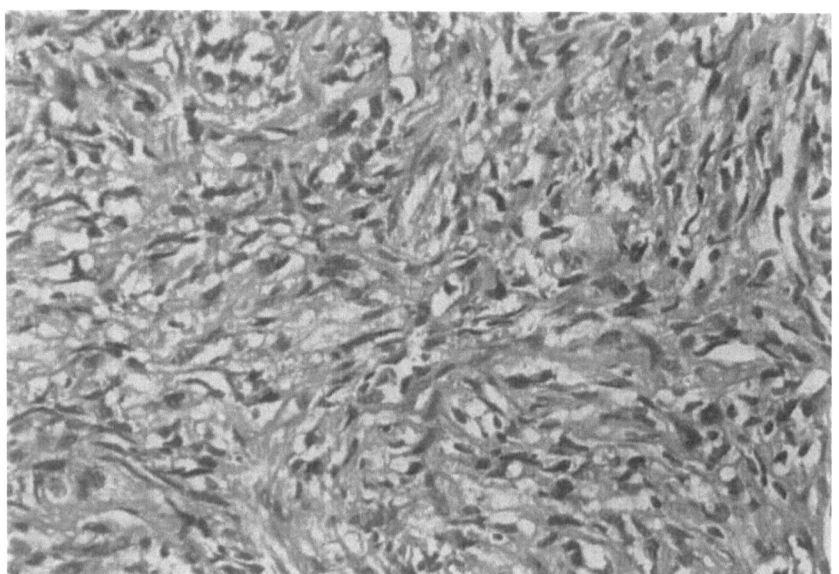

Figure 63 Connective tissue type. A cellular-rich area from the same case as Figure 62 (× 275)

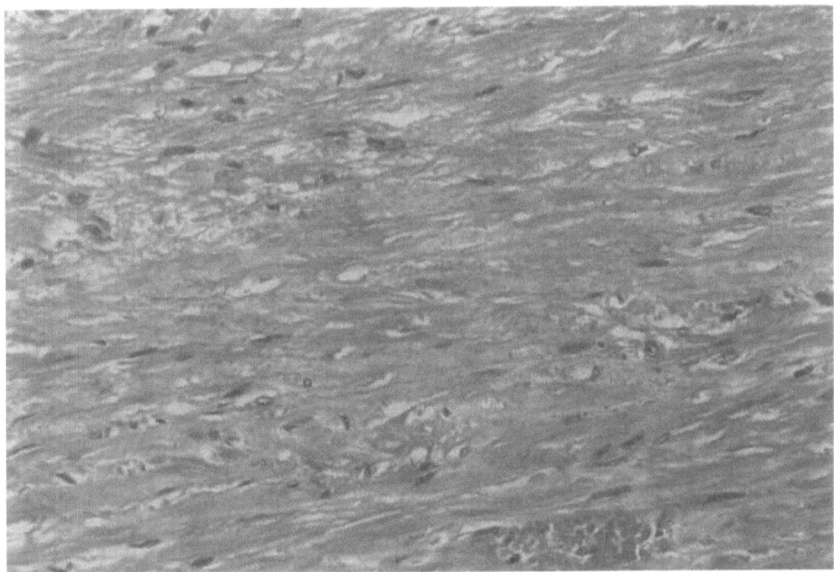

Figure 64 Connective tissue type dominated by collagen. The scanty cells are pleo-morphic (× 275)

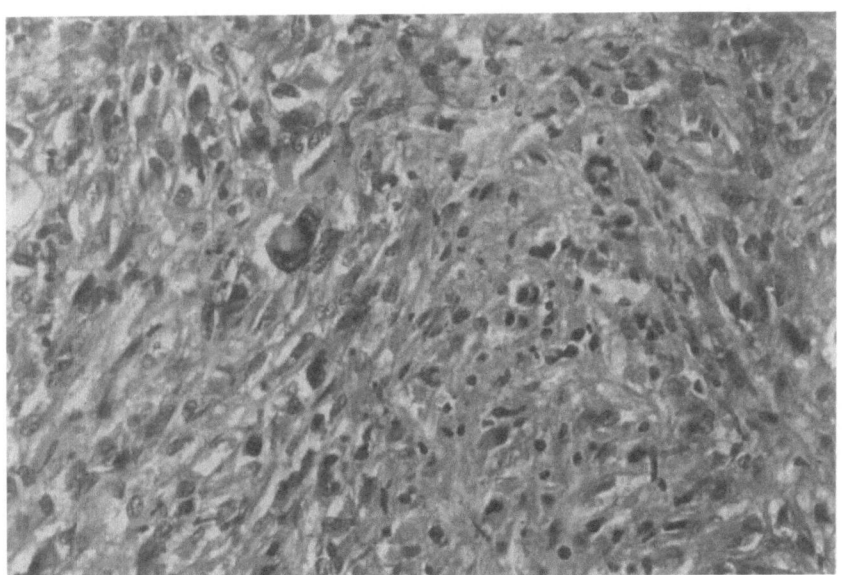

Figure 65 Connective tissue type showing a pleomorphic appearance with multi-nucleated giant cells adjacent to a small area of necrosis (× 275)

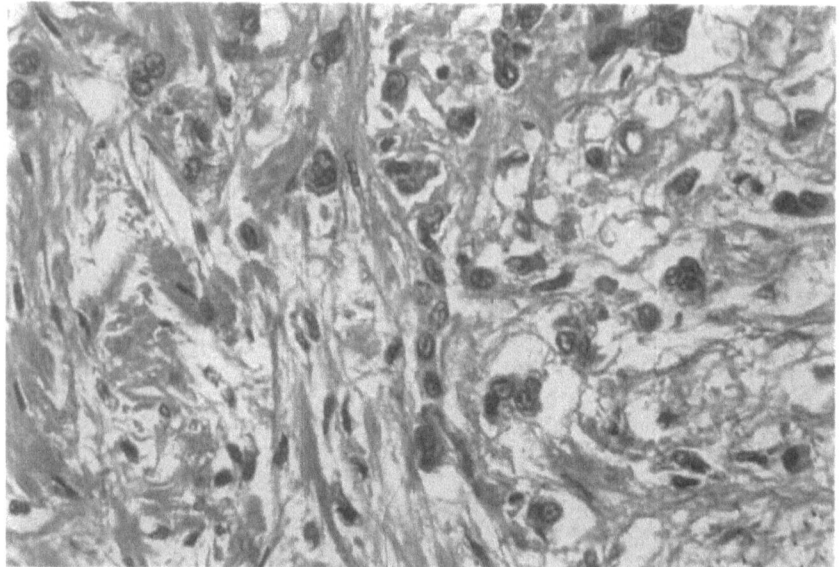

Figure 66 Connective tissue type showing pleomorphic giant cells and irregular collagen bundles (× 430)

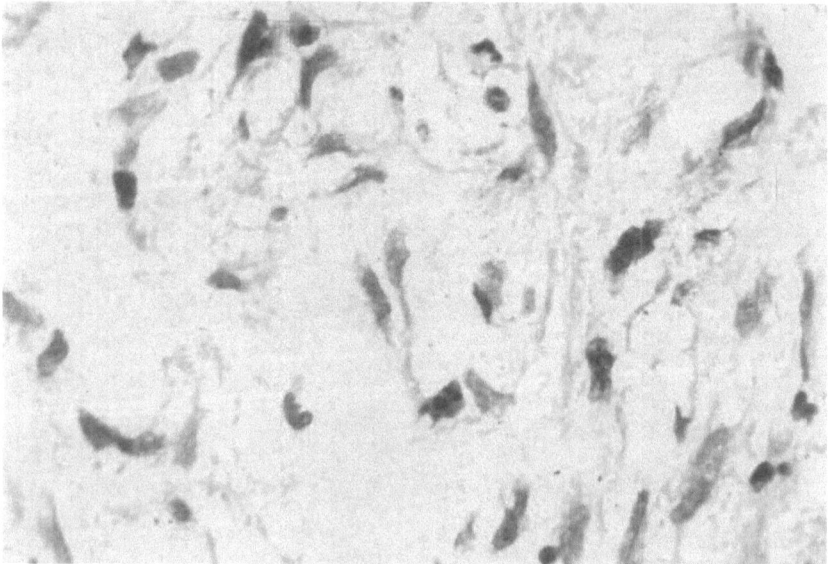

Figure 67 Connective tissue type; high power view, showing pleomorphic cells and loose collagen fibrils (× 730)

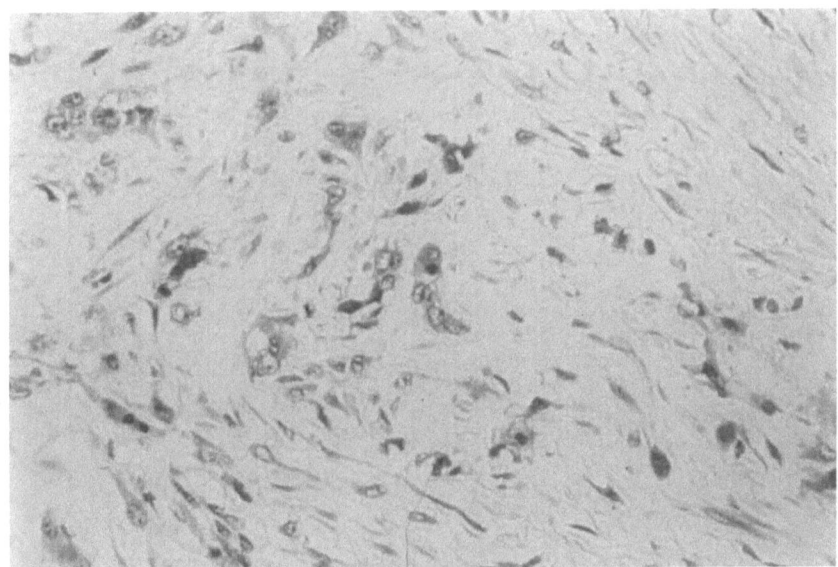

Figure 68 Connective tissue type showing a myxoid appearance (× 275)

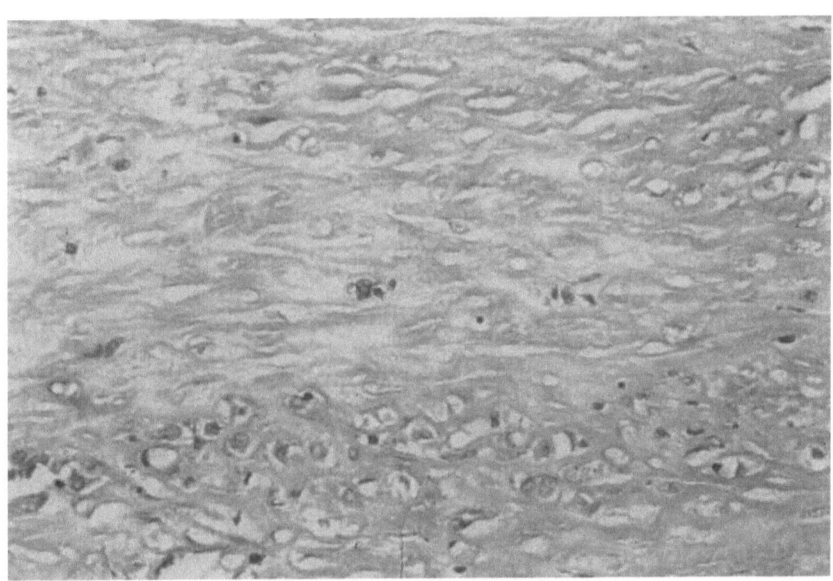

Figure 69 Connective tissue type showing abundant collagen and a chondroid appearance in the lower zone (× 275)

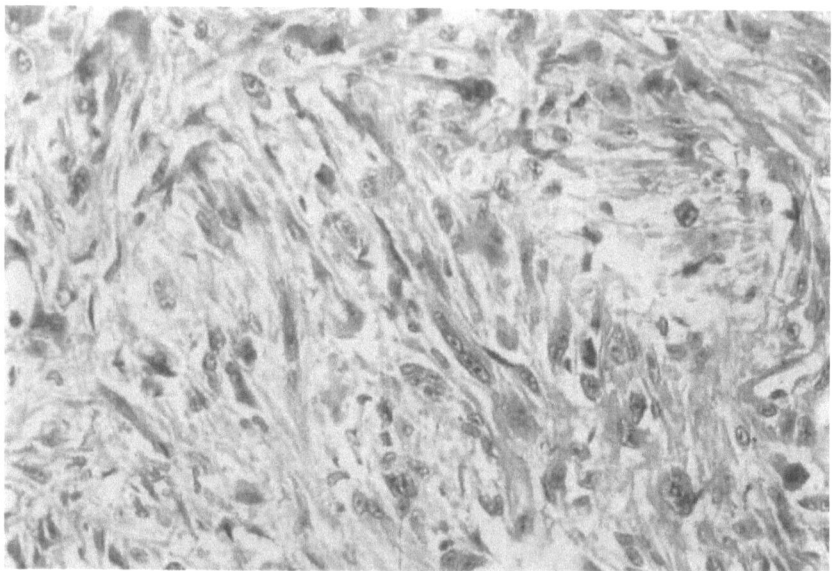

Figure 70   Pleomorphic connective tissue type suggestive of sarcomatous differentiation (× 275)

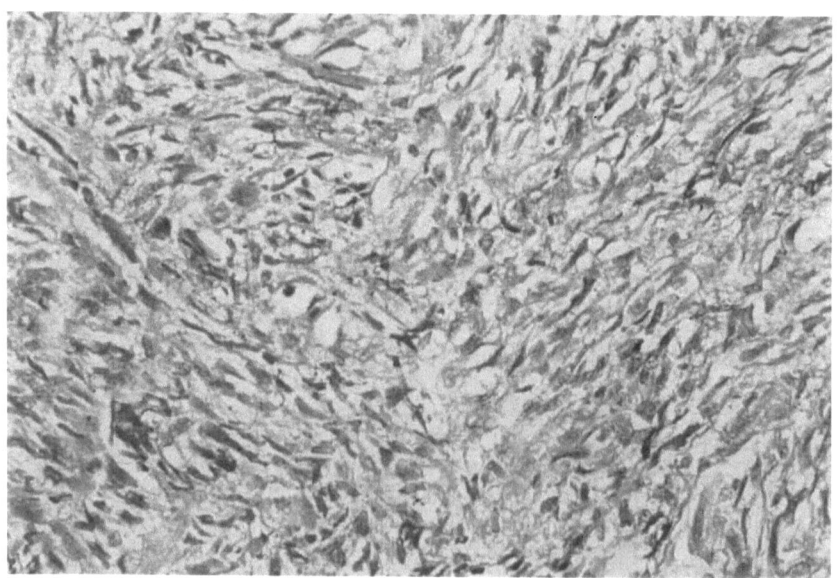

Figure 71   Pleomorphic connective tissue type suggestive of fibro-sarcomatous differentiation. PAS stain (× 275)

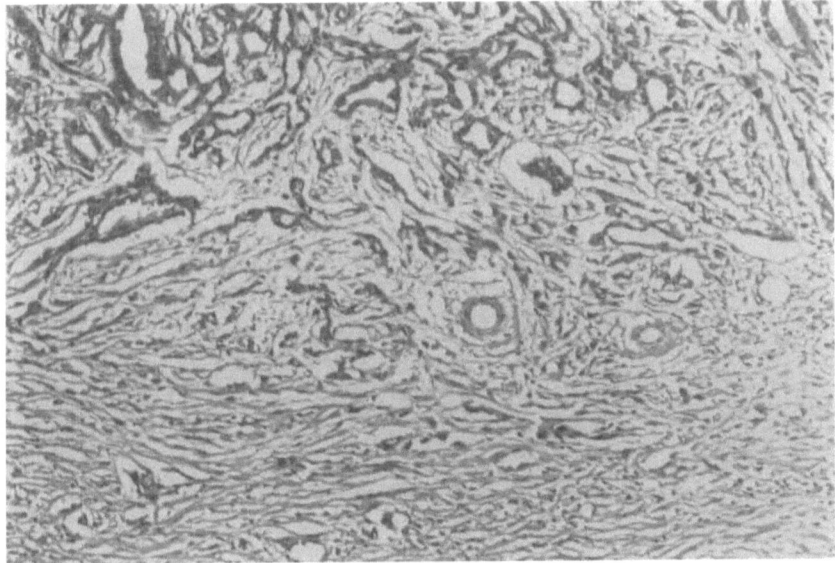

Figure 72 Mixed type with epithelial predominance in the upper zone (× 110)

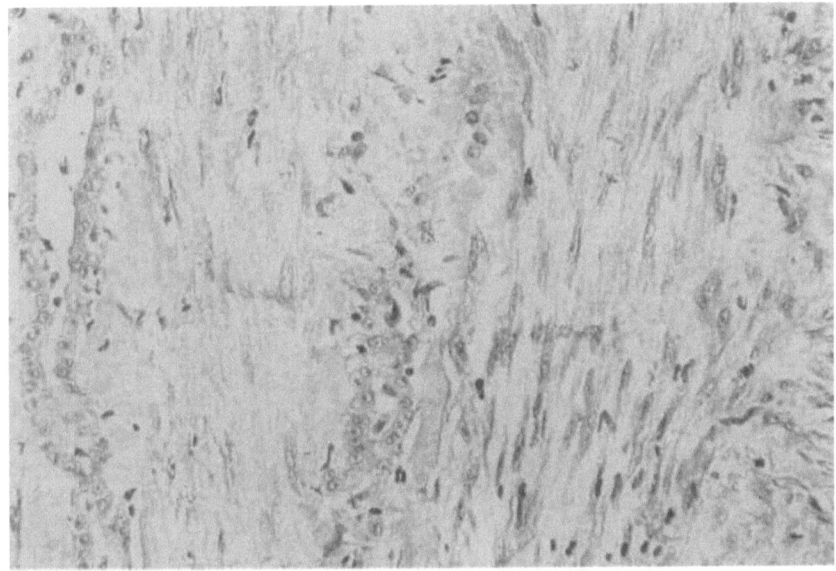

Figure 73 Mixed type with epithelial tubules, collagen and spindle cells (× 275)

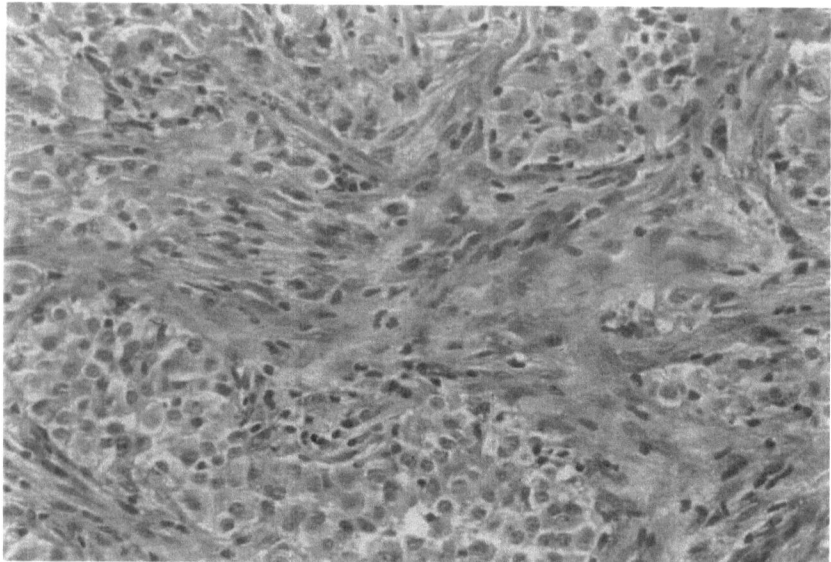

Figure 74   Mixed type. Some of the cell nests are difficult to differentiate between epithelial cells and bundles of spindle cells cut across the longitudinal axis (× 275)

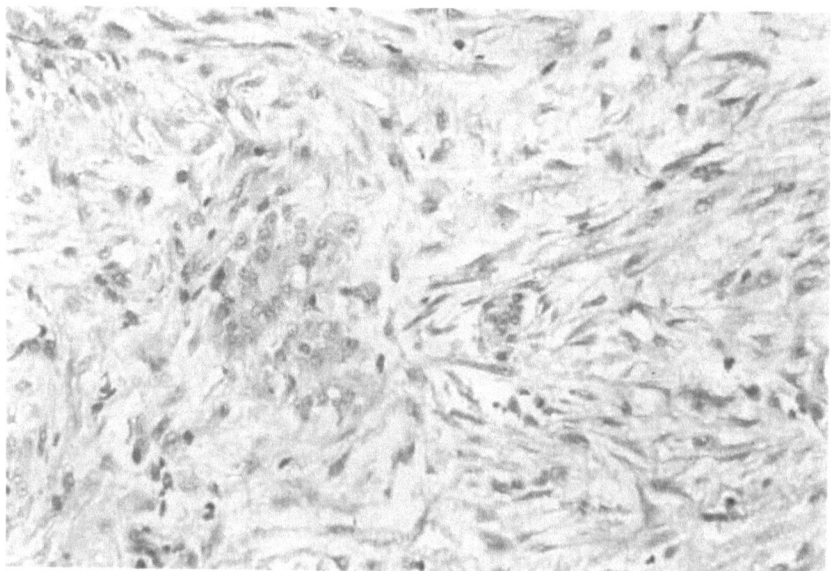

Figure 75   Mixed type with close intermingling between epithelial and connective tissue elements (× 275)

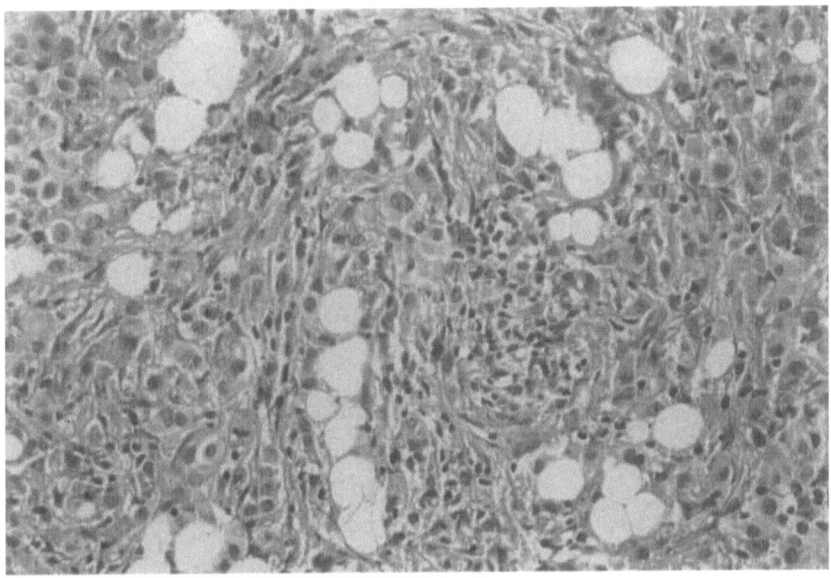

Figure 76 Mixed type invading fatty tissue. Scattered lymphocytes are present (× 275)

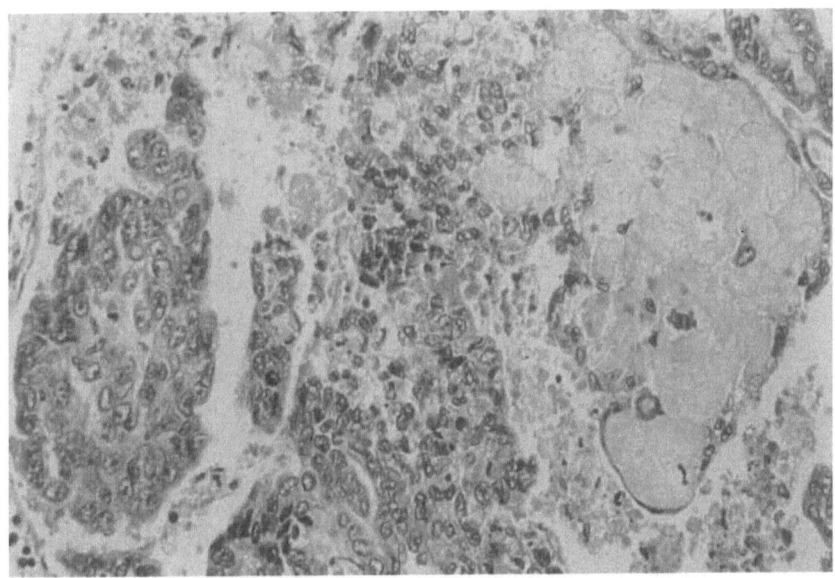

Figure 77 Mainly epithelial type with a deposit of amyloid (× 275)

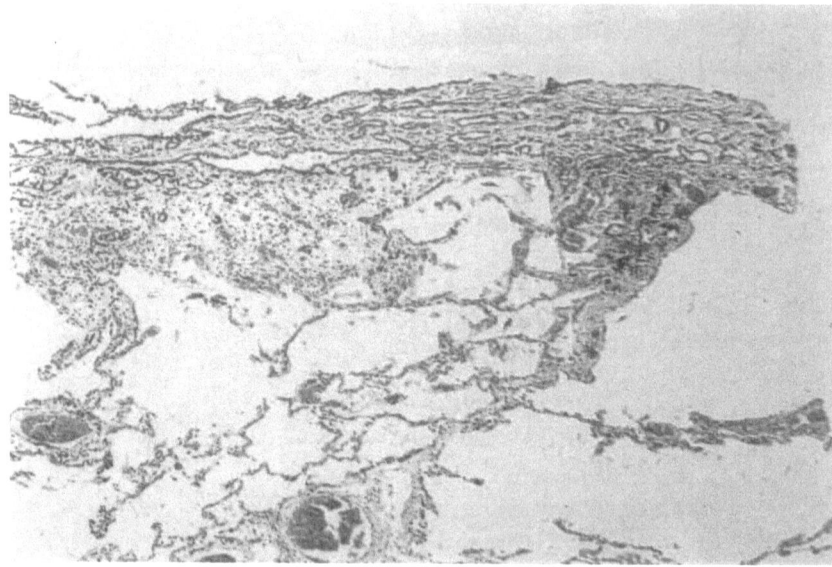

Figure 78 Low power view of a mesothelioma of the pleura of mainly epithelial type which presented macroscopically as a small area of thickened visceral pleura, indistinguishable from non-specific fibrosis. This specimen came from a patient with a carcinoma of the bronchus and asbestosis (× 45) (This case was kindly contributed by Dr W.S. Kwee.)

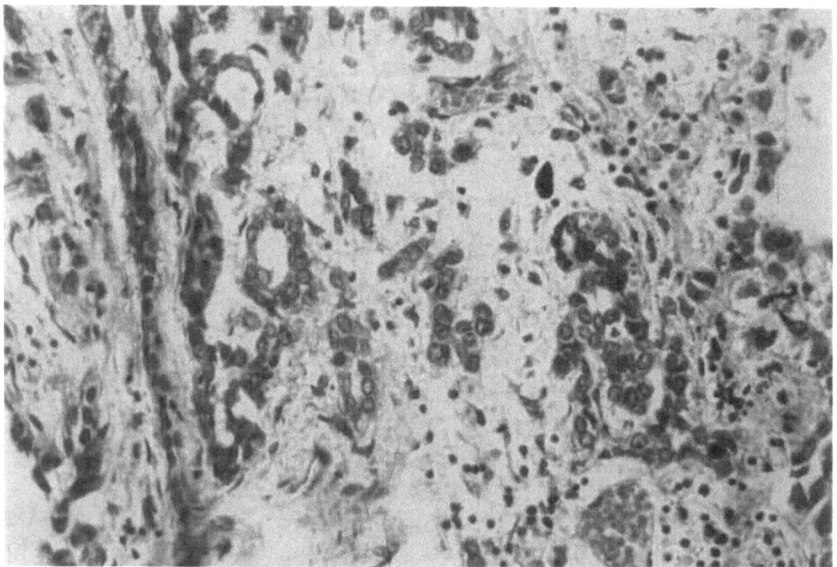

Figure 79 Higher magnification of Figure 78 shows a typical mesothelioma (× 275)

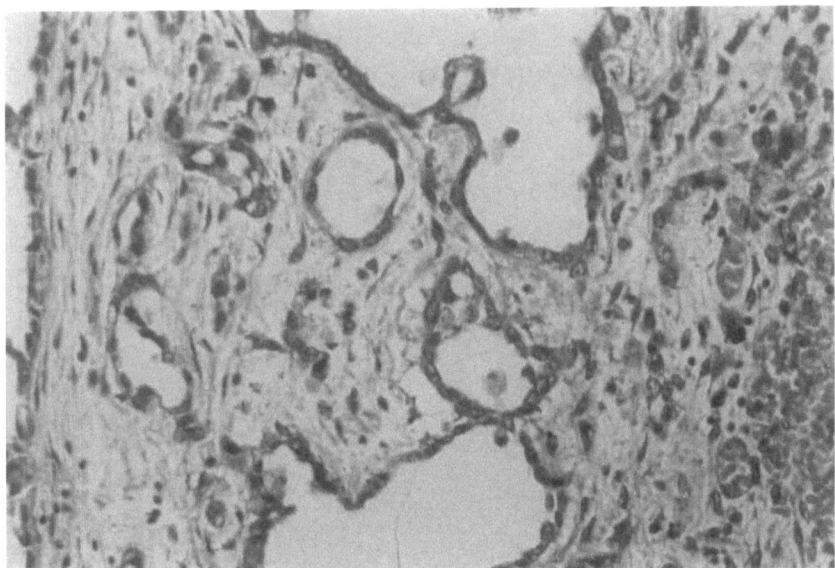

Figure 80   Further view of Figure 78 (× 275)

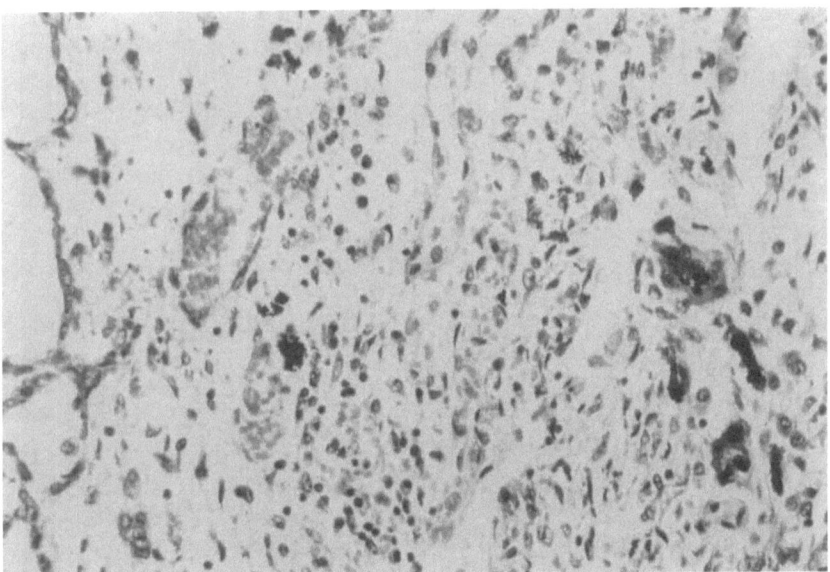

Figure 81   Further view of Figure 78 shows epithelial type mesothelioma on the left side. The darkly staining structures on the right side are asbestos bodies which are present in the peripheral lung tissue (× 275)

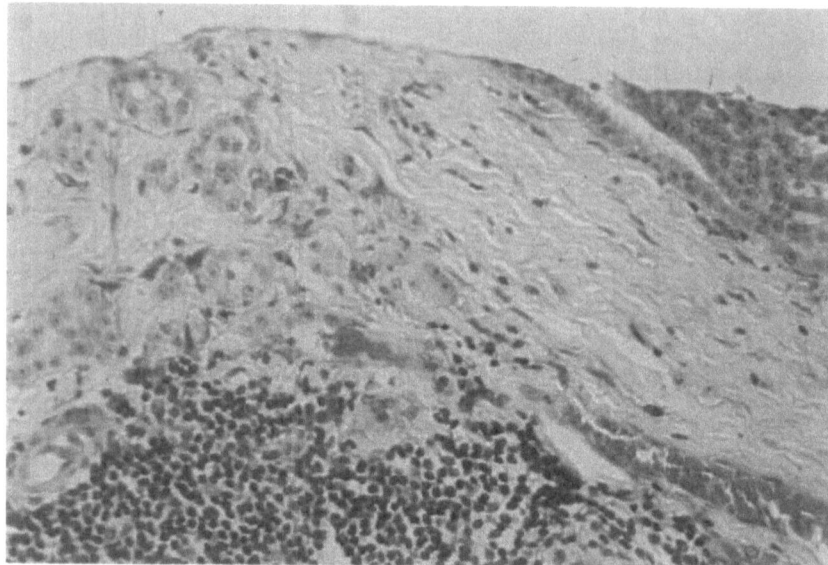

Figure 82 A single layer of flattened mesothelial cells at the top of the picture shows changes of hyperplasia and neoplasia in the top right hand corner. In the thickened sub-mesothelial tissue there are tubules of epithelial type mesothelioma. There is lymphocytic infiltration at the bottom (× 275)

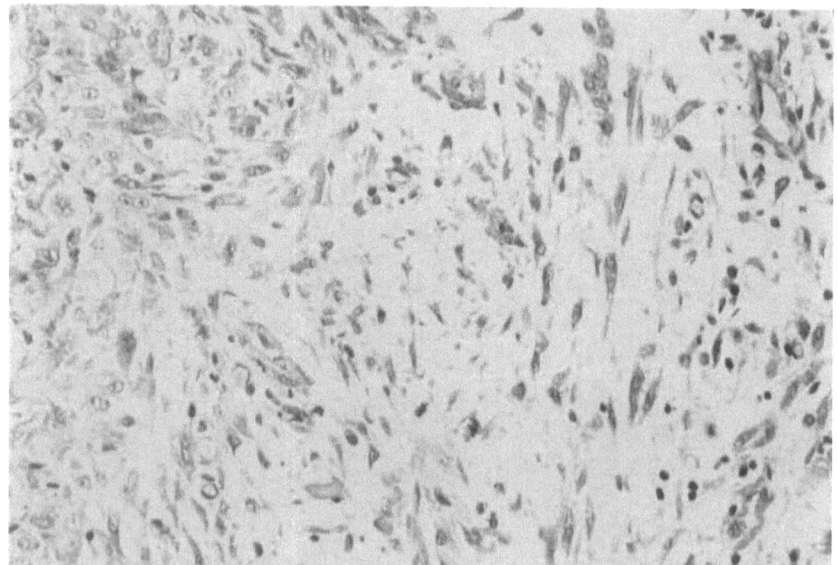

Figure 83 Another site from the same tumour as in Figure 82, showing a mixed type of mesothelioma (× 275)

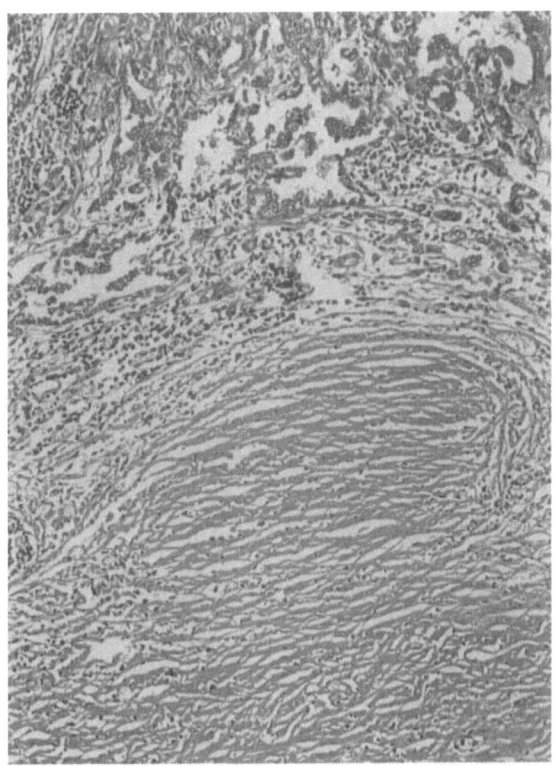

Figure 84 An epithelial type of mesothelioma of tubulo-papillary pattern on the surface of a pleural plaque (× 110)

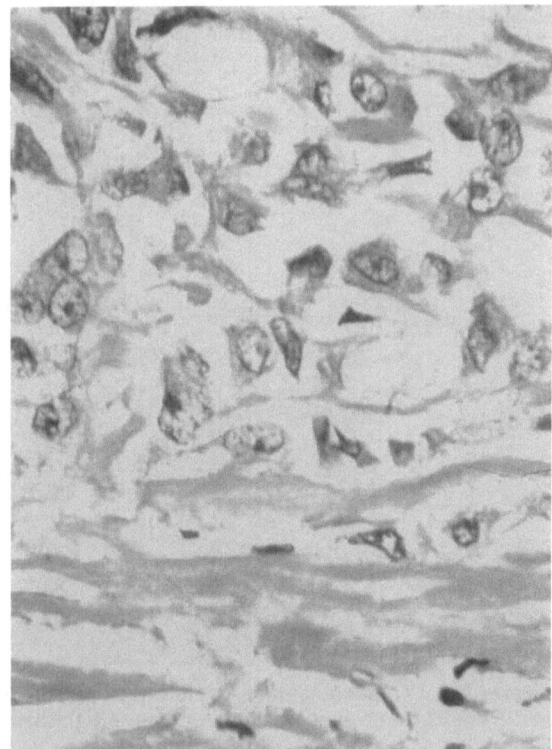

Figure 85 A high power view of the above section (× 730)

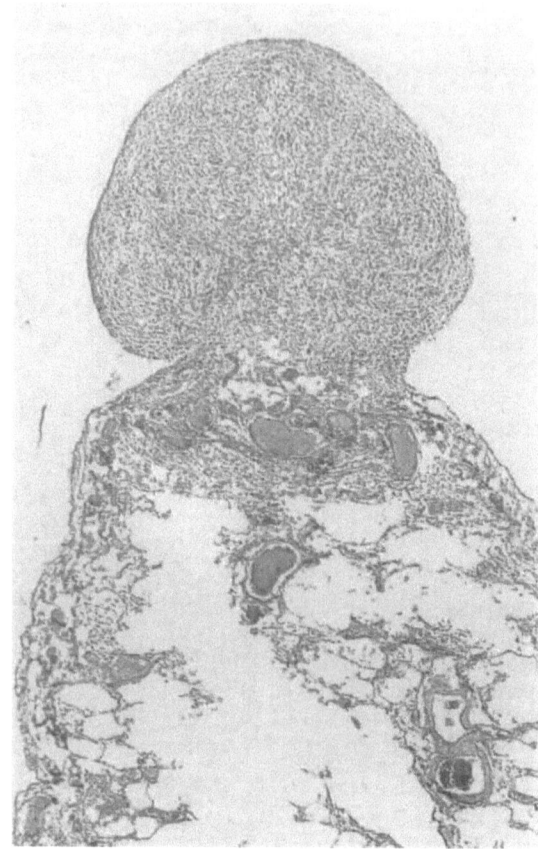

Figure 86   A metastatic nodule of mesothelioma on the visceral pleura from a primary mesothelioma of the peritoneum (× 25)

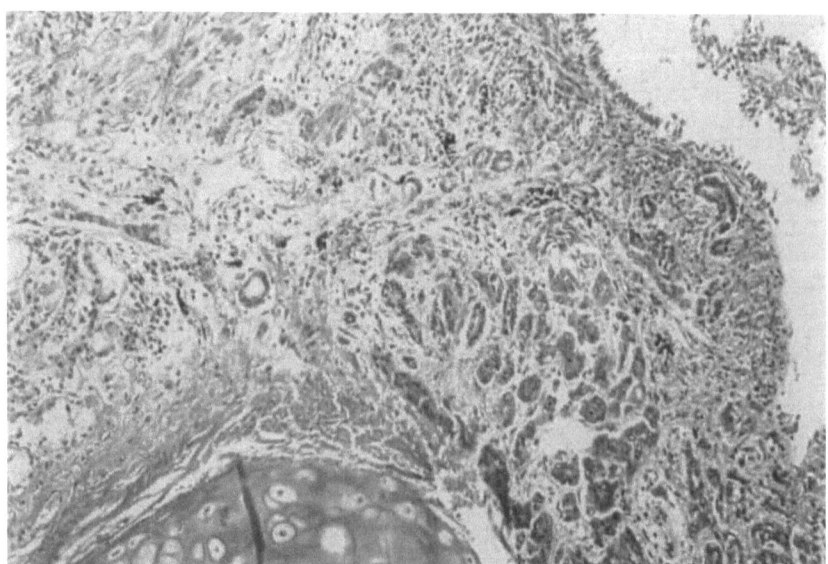

Figure 87   Lymphatic spread of mesothelioma in the bronchial wall. Note the partly intact bronchial epithelium in the top right hand corner (× 110)

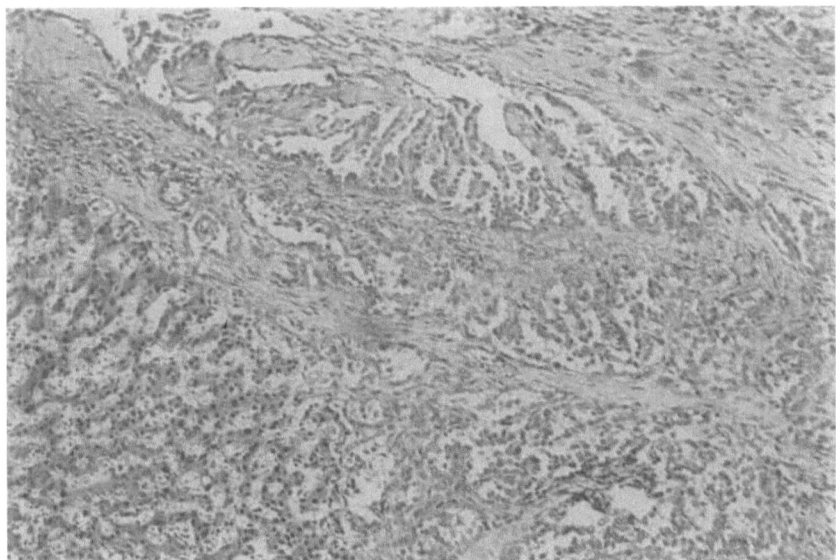

Figure 88 Mesothelioma of the peritoneum, epithelial type, with a tubulo-papillary pattern. There is shallow infiltration into the liver capsule and parenchyma (× 110)

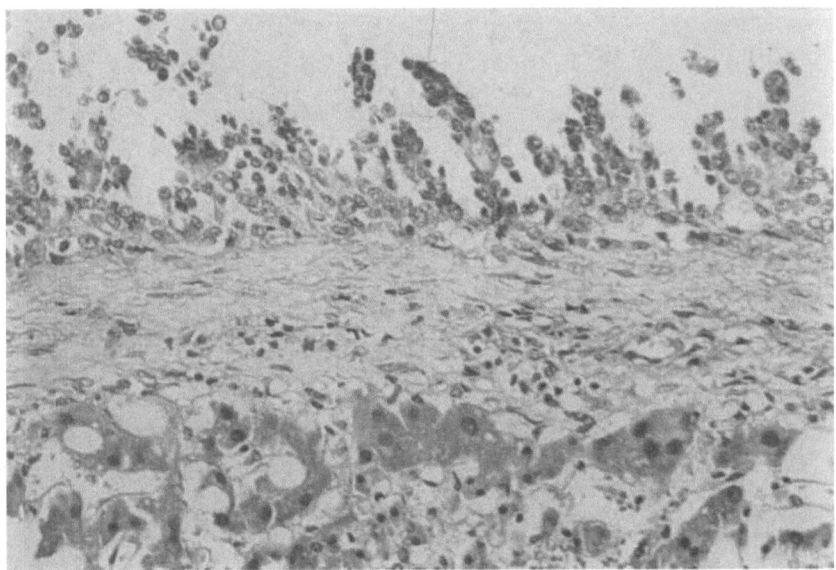

Figure 89   A higher power view of the same case as in Figure 88 (× 275)

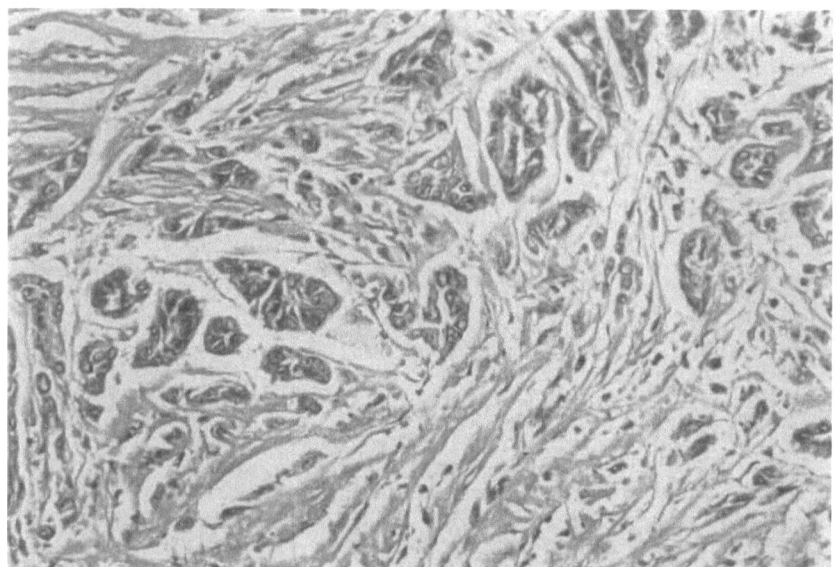

Figure 90   A mixed type of mesothelioma invading connective tissue (× 275)

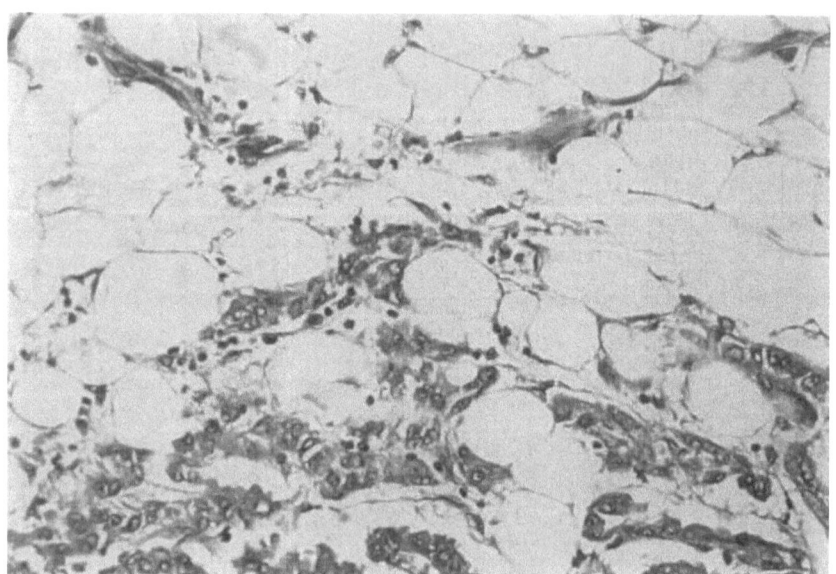

Figure 91   A mainly epithelial area in a mixed type of mesothelioma which is invading fat (× 275)

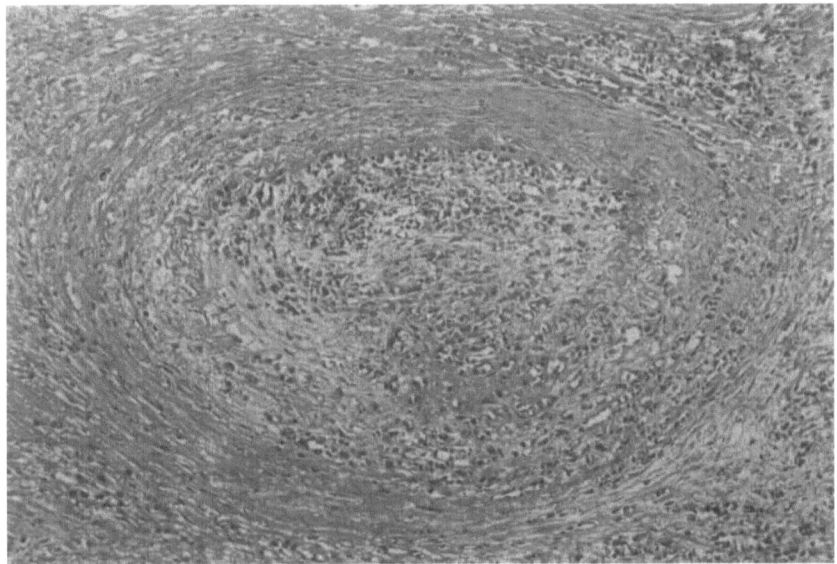

Figure 92 A mesothelioma destroying the wall, and obstructing the lumen of an artery (× 110)

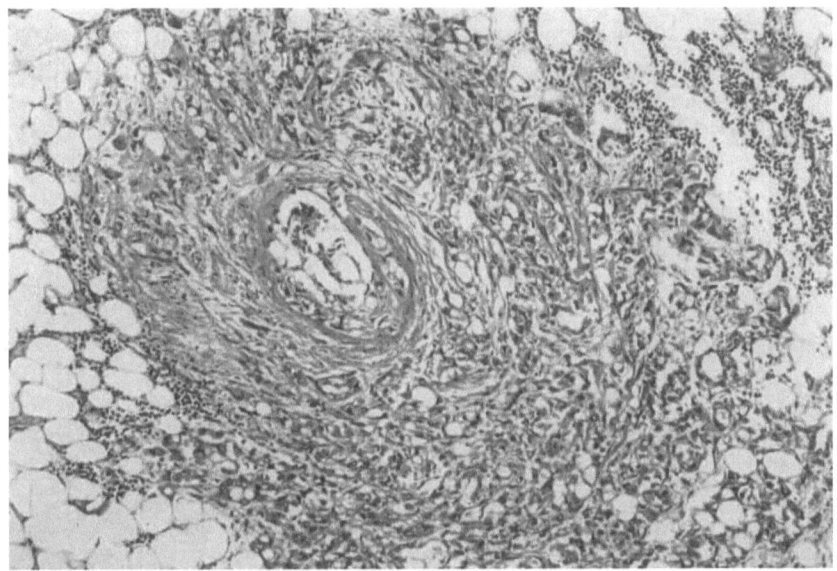

Figure 93 Spread of a mesothelioma which is predominantly perivascular, but which also involves the wall and lumen of the vein (× 110)

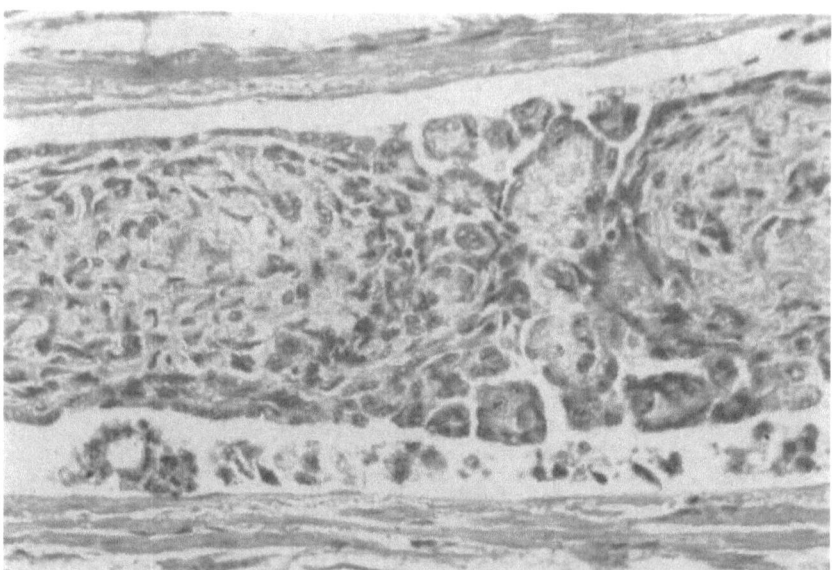

Figure 94   A mixed type of mesothelioma causing obstruction of the lumen of a vein without involvement of the vessel wall (× 275)

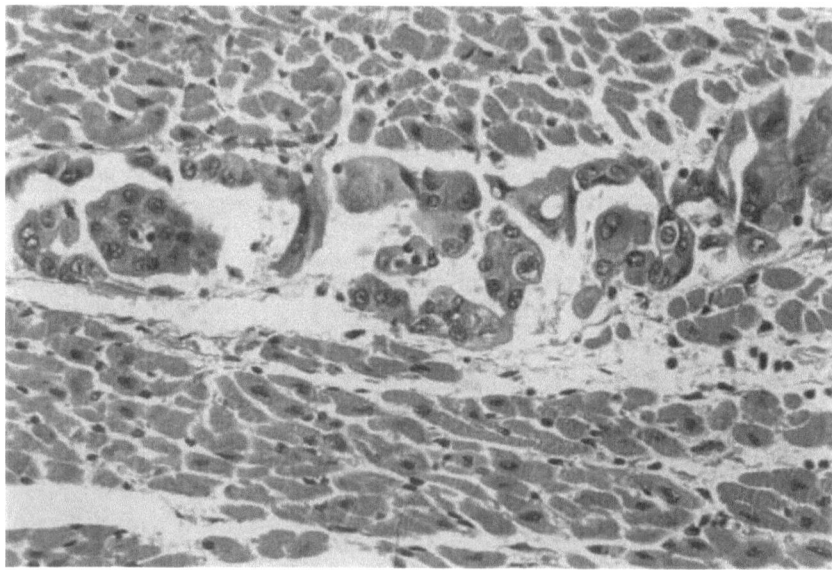

Figure 95   An epithelial type of mesothelioma spreading within the myocardium (× 275)

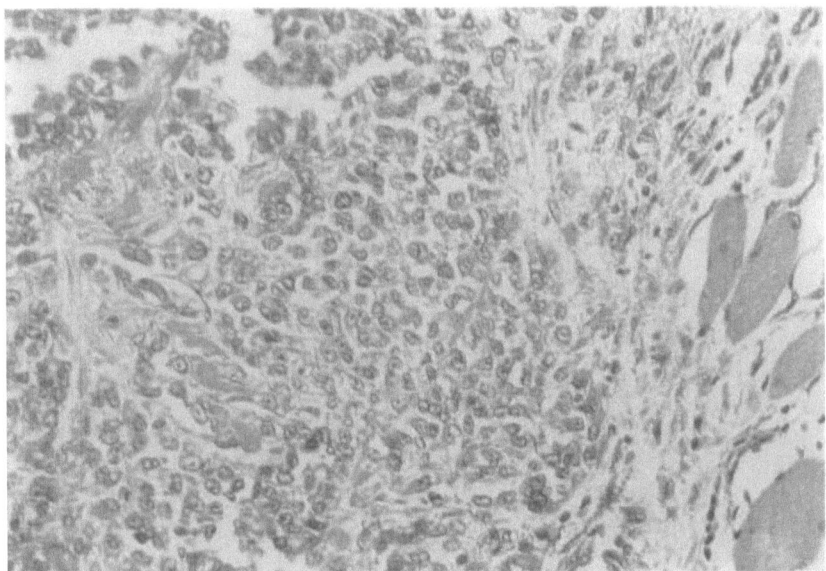

Figure 96 A mixed type of mesothelioma invading the intercostal muscle at the site of thoracoscopy which had been performed several months earlier (× 275)

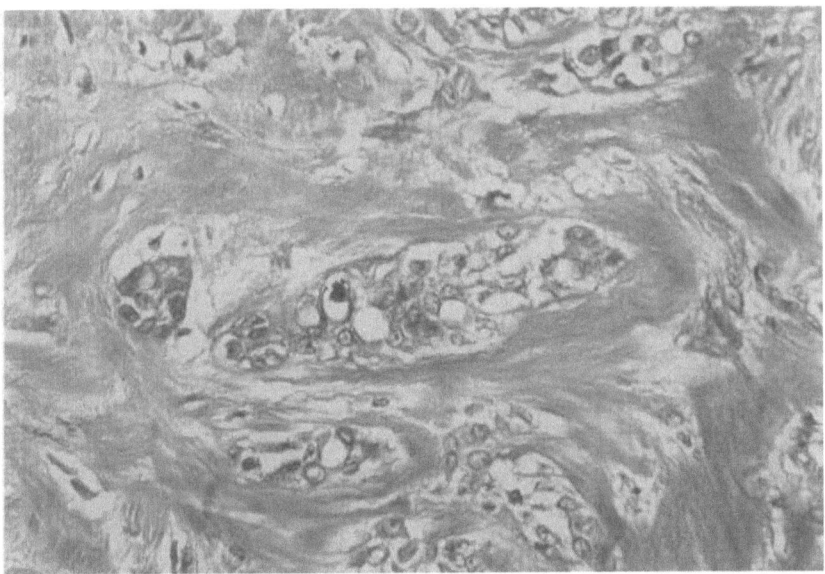

Figure 97 Tumour within subcutaneous scar tissue from the same case as above but removed 9 months later (× 275)

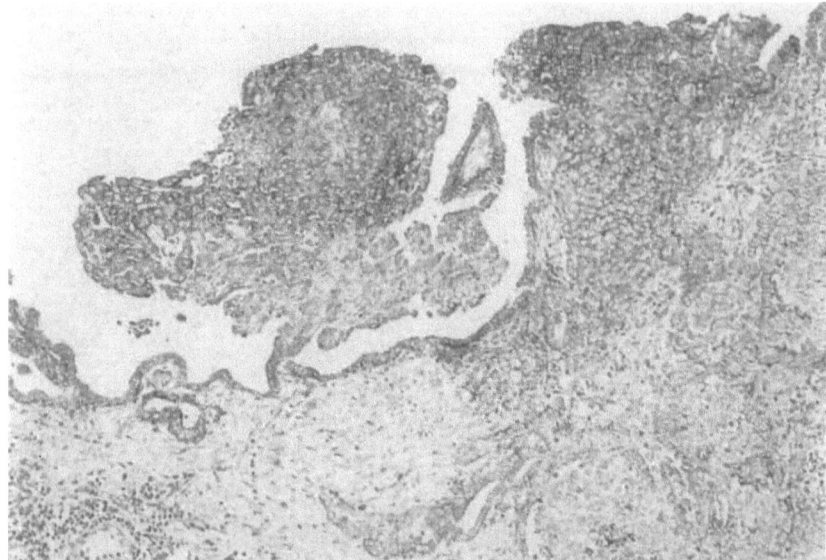

Figure 98 A typical mesothelioma in which the glycogen has stained positively with PAS (× 110)

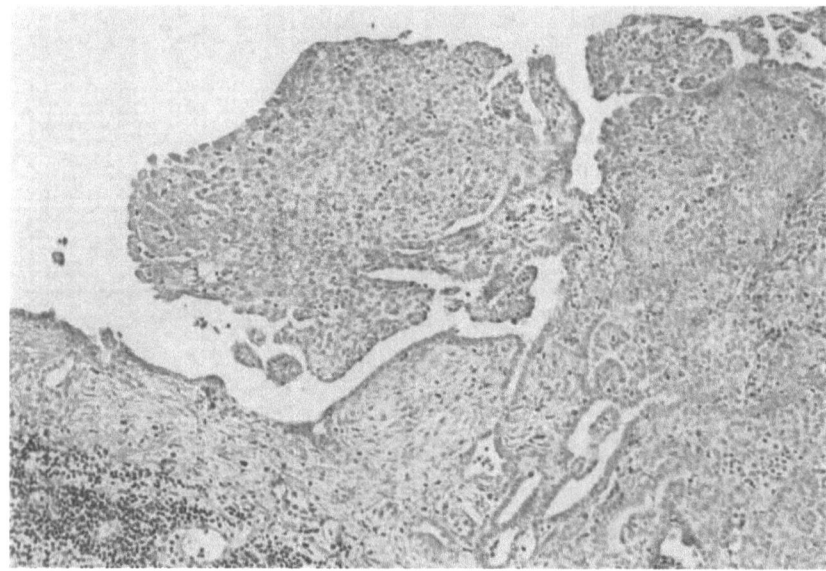

Figure 99 The same case as in Figure 98. The PAS–positive material has been removed by pretreatment with diastase (× 110)

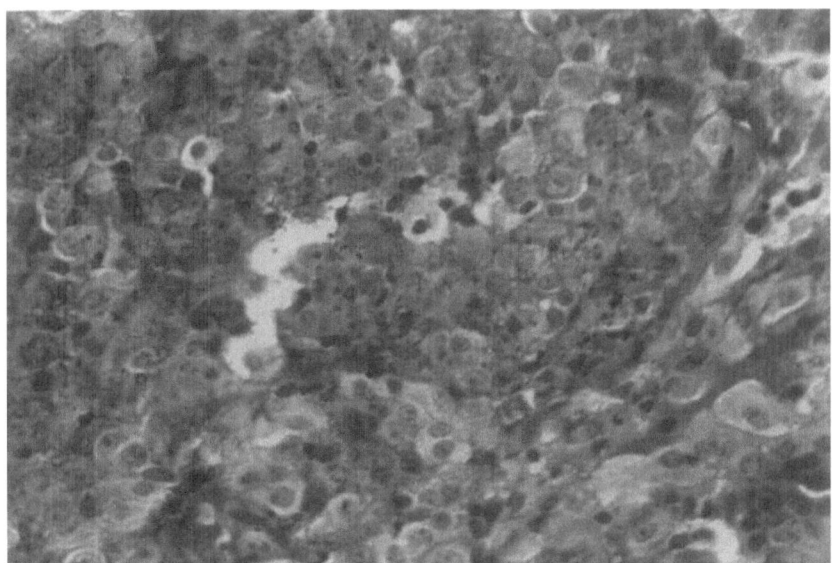

Figure 100   Solid sheets of epithelial type cells from a mesothelioma which have stained positively with PAS (× 430)

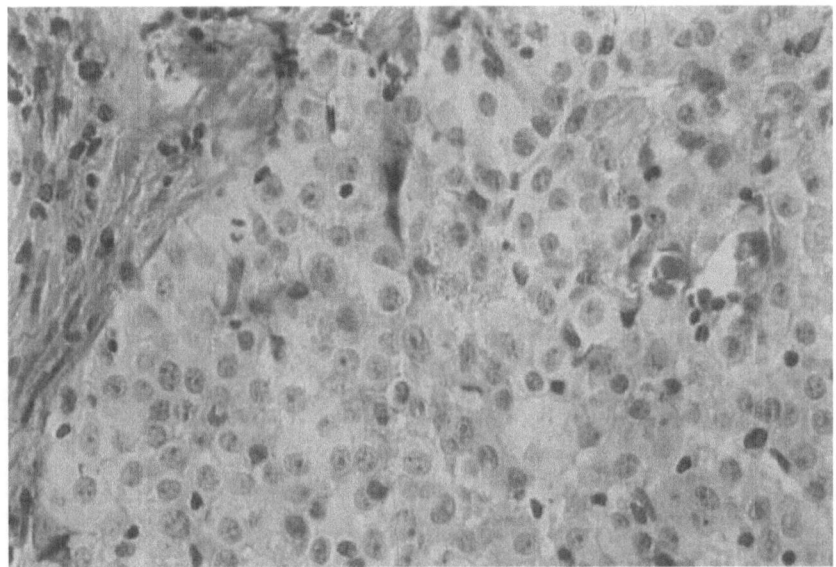

Figure 101   The same case as in Figure 100. The PAS–positive material has been removed by pretreatment with diastase, except for a few fine granules in the centre of the picture. The two positively stained spots on the right are extra-cellular (× 430)

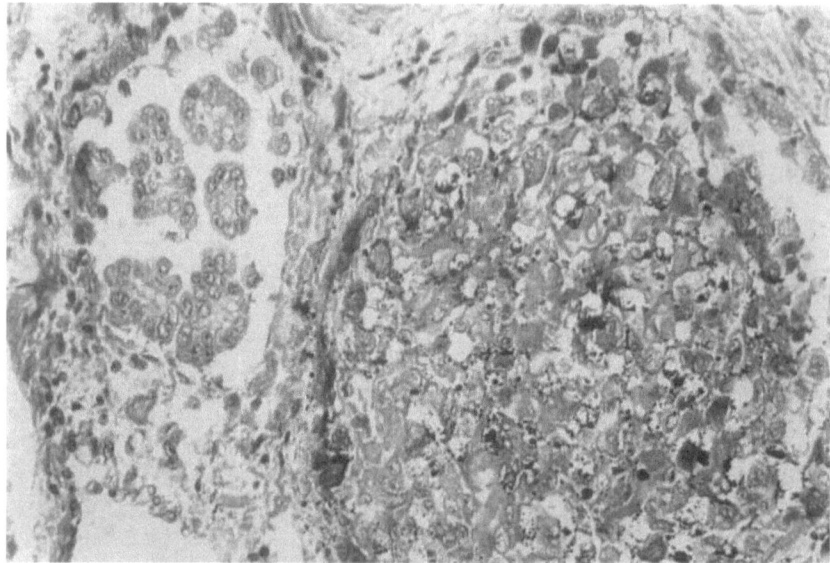

Figure 102 An epithelial type of mesothelioma consisting of a solid sheet of cells which are PAS–positive. The papillary cells within the lymphatic vessel are PAS–negative (× 275)

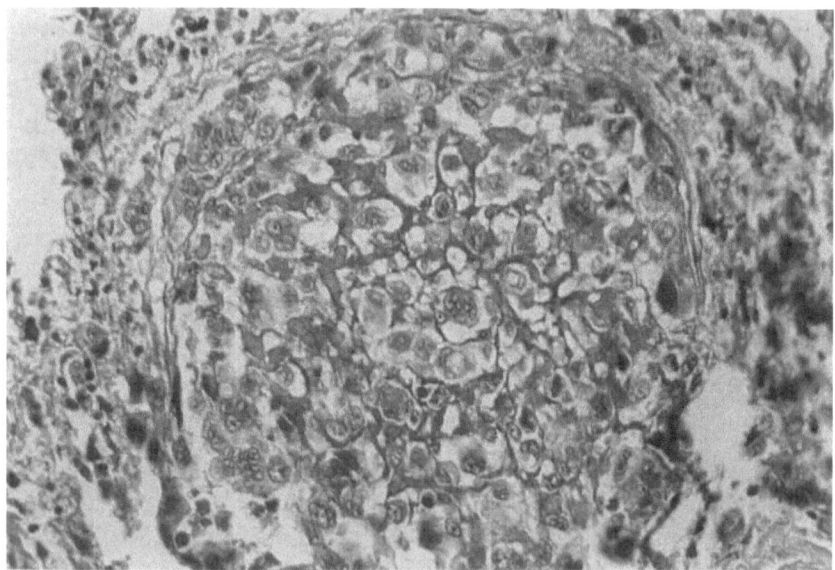

Figure 103 The solid sheet of cells in the above section shows negative staining of the individual cells with diastase–PAS, but positive staining of the intercellular substance (× 275)

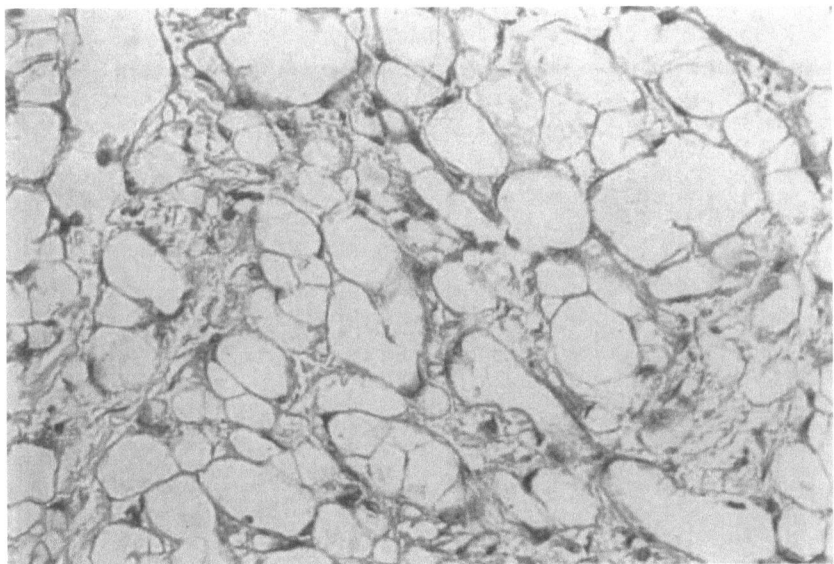

Figure 104   Epithelial type, tubular pattern with a microcystic appearance. This is the same case as in Figure 50. This section suggests a liposarcomatous differentiation on H & E staining (× 275)

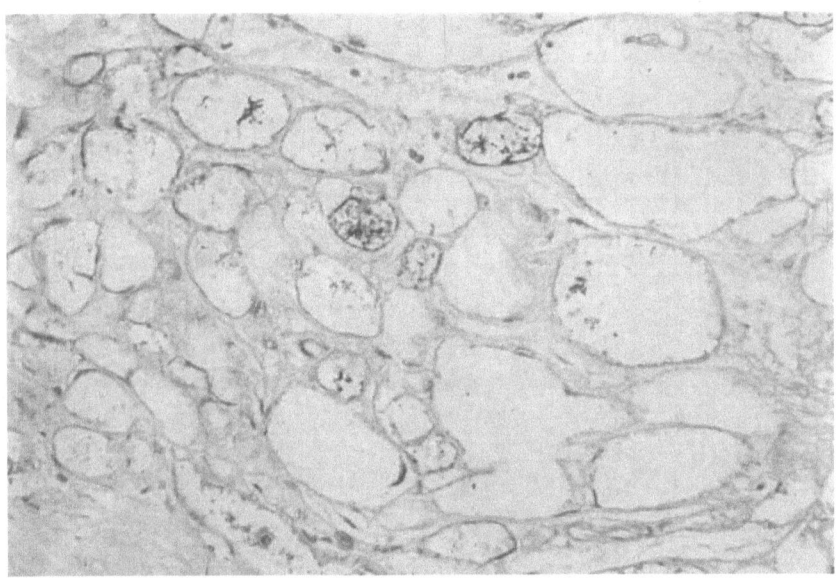

Figure 105   The alcian blue stain is positive, indicating the presence of mucopolysaccharides in the cystic spaces. This is in keeping with the diagnosis of mesothelioma (× 275)

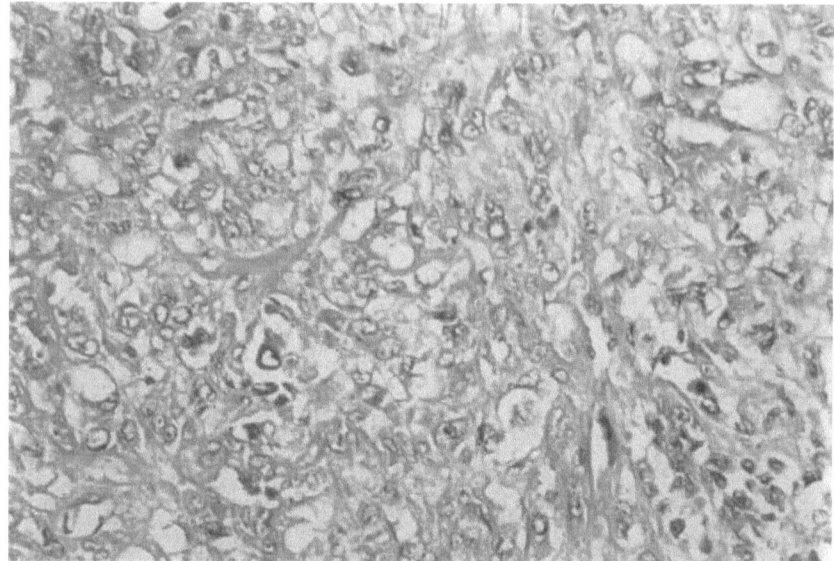

Figure 106   A poorly differentiated mixed type of mesothelioma. This section suggests the possibility of an undifferentiated carcinoma (× 275)

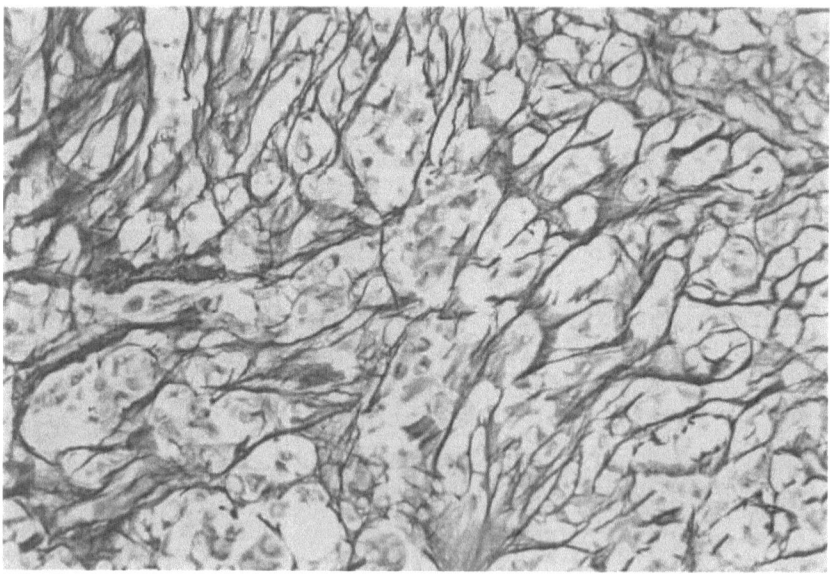

Figure 107   The Gomori reticulin stain of the above section shows a more intimate framework of reticulin around the tumour cells than would be expected in a carcinoma (× 275)

Cytology of effusions

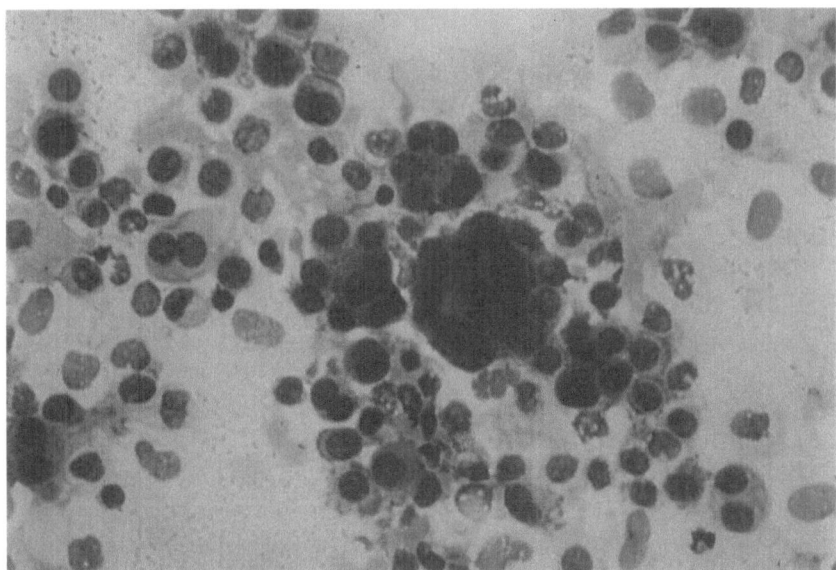

Figure 108 'Raspberry' form of papillary epithelial type surrounded by single mesothelial cells to demonstrate the general cellular pattern. Jenner-Giemsa stain (× 400)

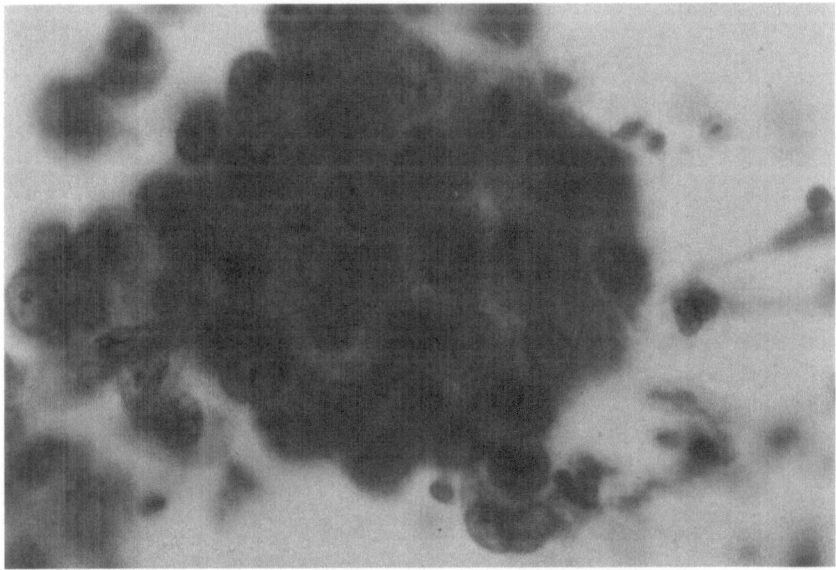

Figure 109 A higher magnification of a similar structure to show the 'raspberry' formation. Papanicolaou stain (× 800)

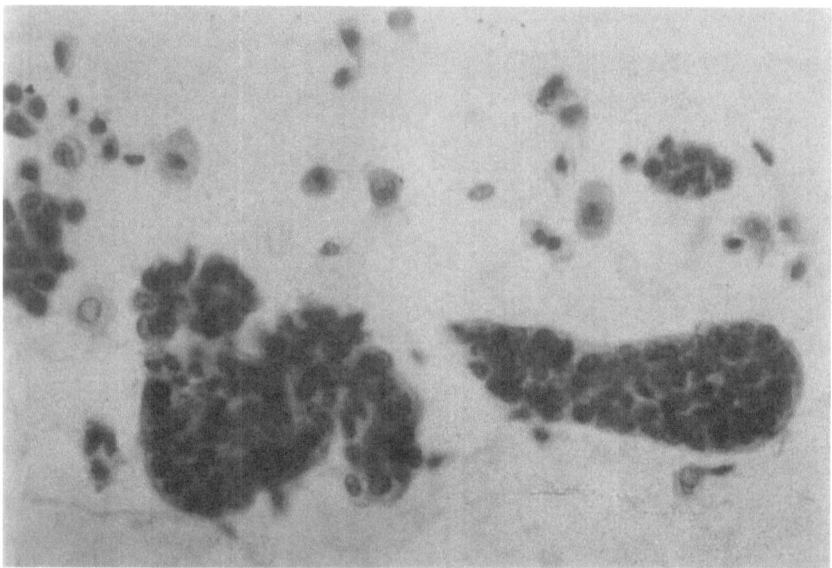

Figure 110   Epithelial type of mesothelioma to show tubular structure in the smear sample. Papanicolaou stain (× 400)

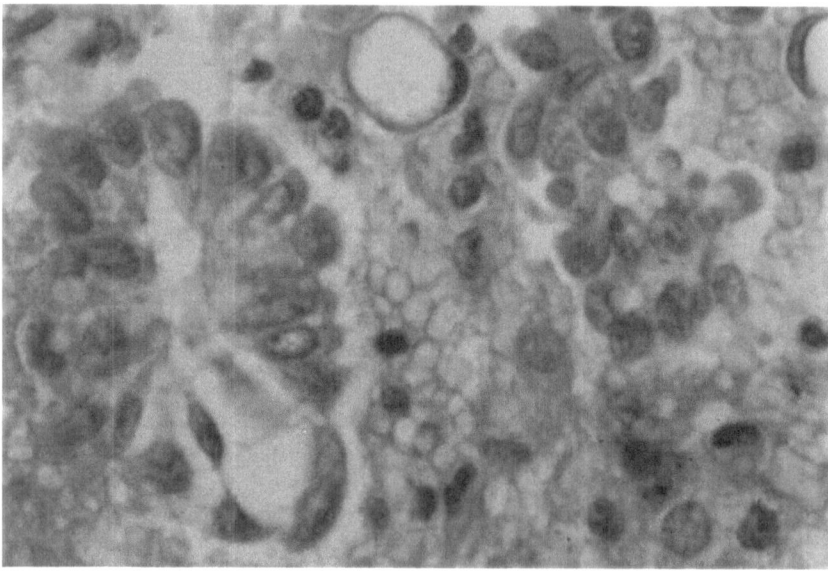

Figure 111   Paraffin section of cell deposit from a similar case to show the tubular structure of an epithelial type of mesothelioma. Single malignant mesothelial cells occupy the rest of the field (× 800)

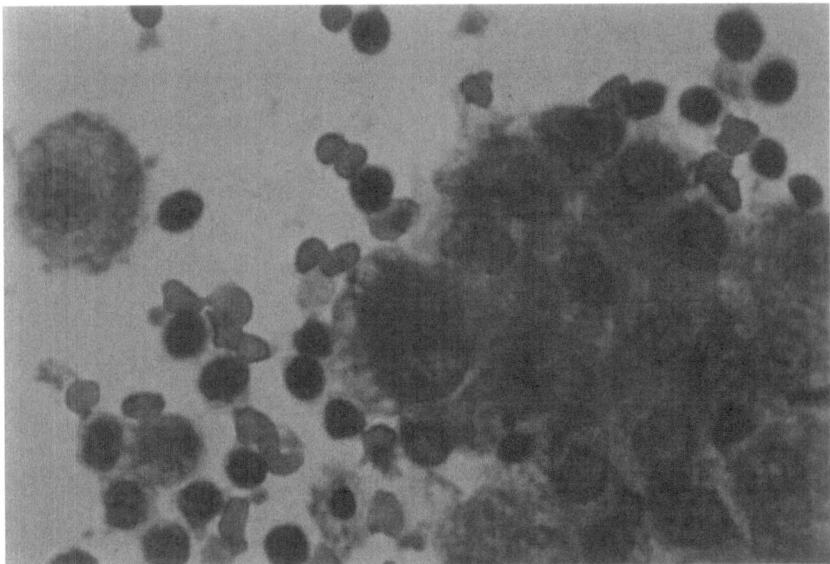

Figure 112   A group of loosely adherent malignant mesothelial cells are seen in one half of the field. These are in contrast to the single reactive mesothelial cell which is isolated in the other half of the field. Papanicolaou stain (× 800)

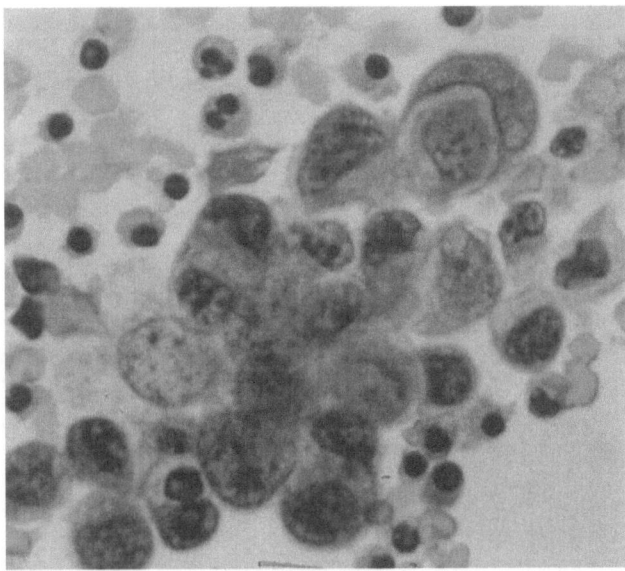

Figure 113   A loose group of malignant mesothelial cells which show pleomorphism and 'pseudo-cannibalism'. Papanicolaou stain (× 800)

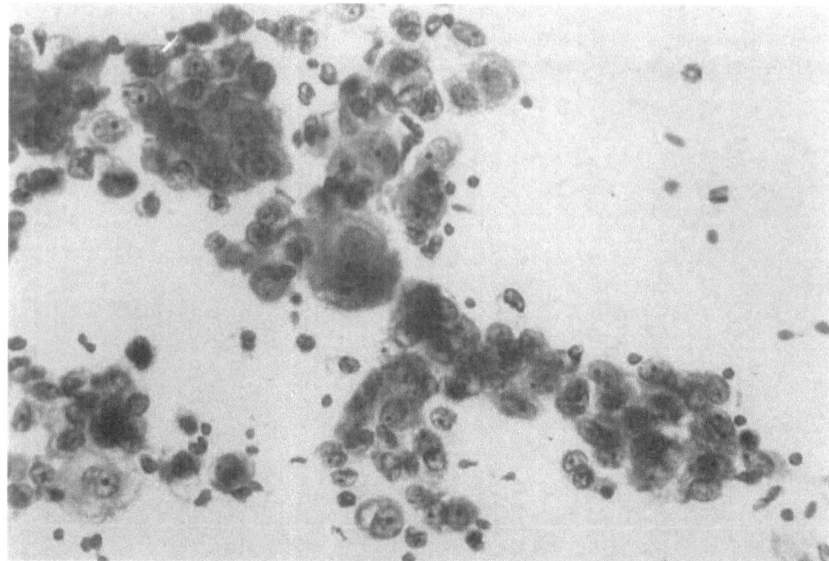

Figure 114 'Raspberry' form of malignant mesothelial cell together with loose chains of cells which show little variation in nuclear or cellular size. Papanicolaou stain (× 400)

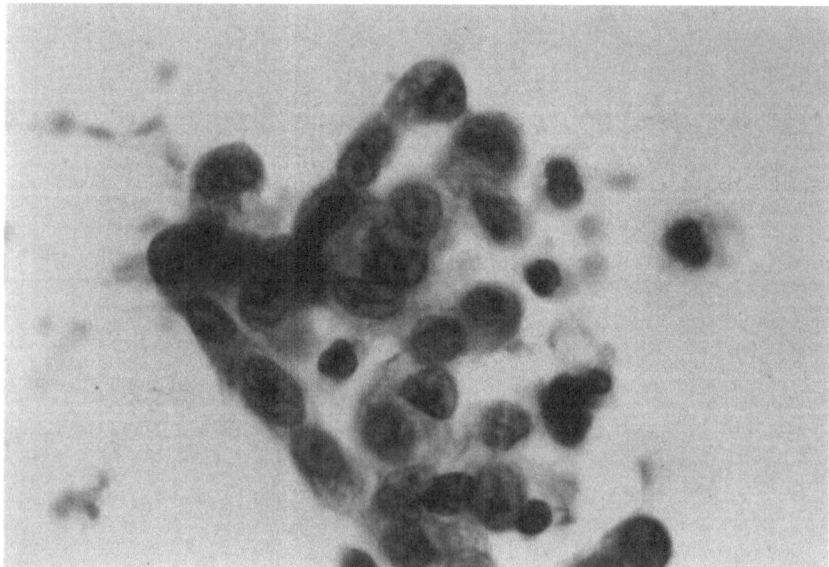

Figure 115   Chains of small malignant mesothelial cells showing little pleomorphism. Papanicolaou stain (× 800)

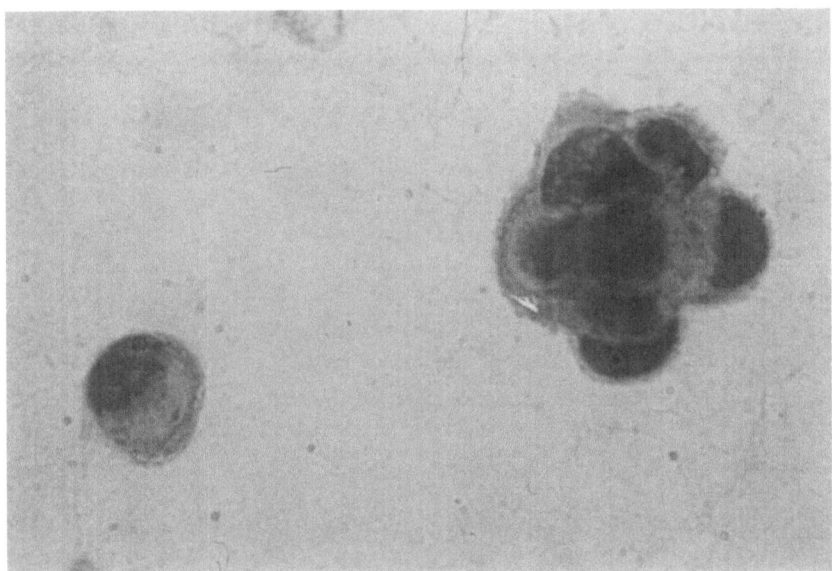

Figure 116   A cluster and an isolated cell of malignant mesothelioma origin. Papanicolaou stain (× 1100)

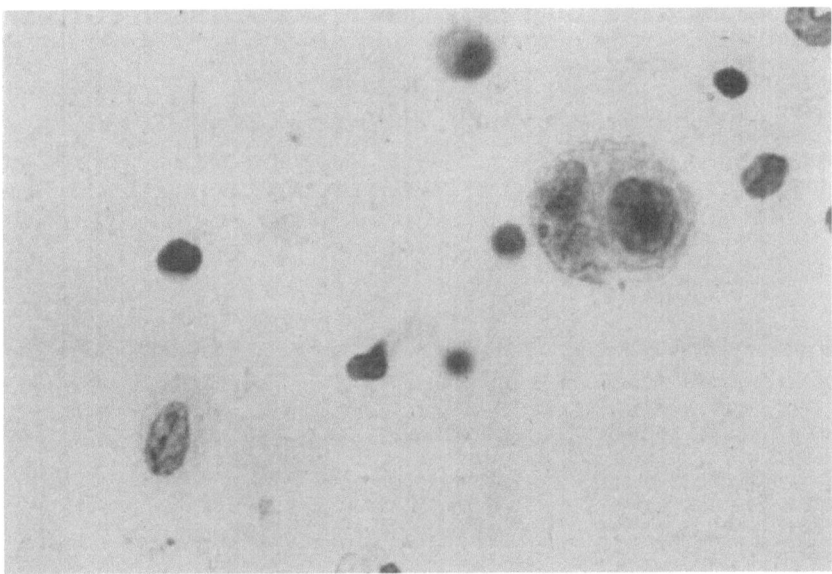

Figure 117   Another field from the above case showing 'pseudo-cannibalism'. Papanicolaou stain (× 1100)

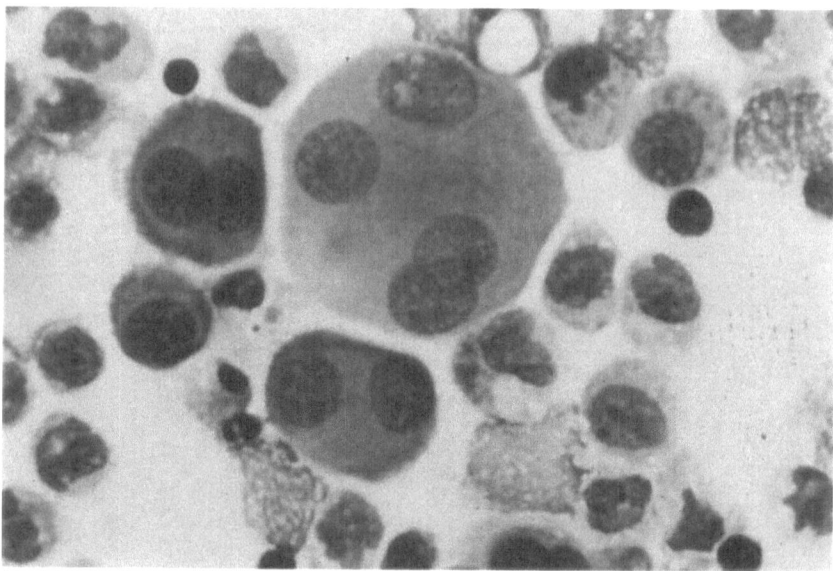

Figure 118   Binucleate and multinucleate malignant mesothelial cells. These cells are larger than those seen in a wet fixed preparation. Jenner-Giemsa stain (× 800)

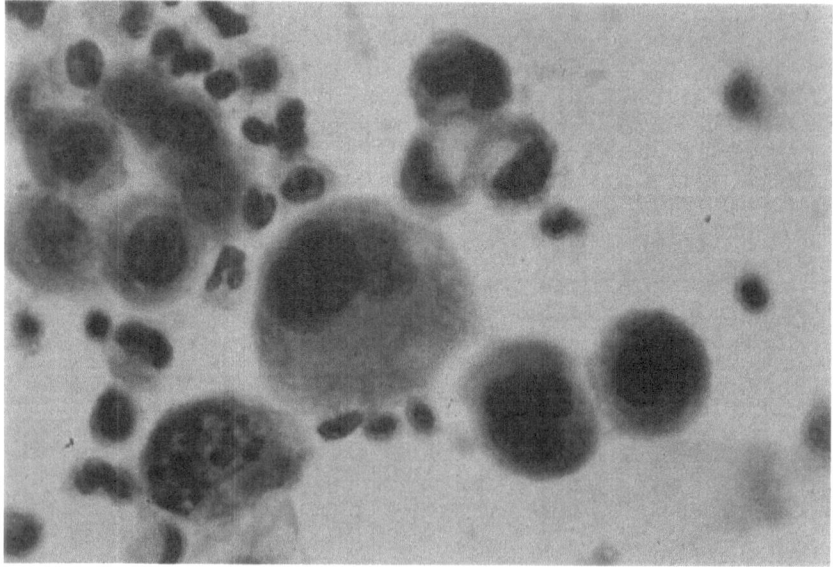

Figure 119   Note the contrast to the above with a wet-fixed Papanicolaou's stain preparation. Papanicolaou stain (× 800)

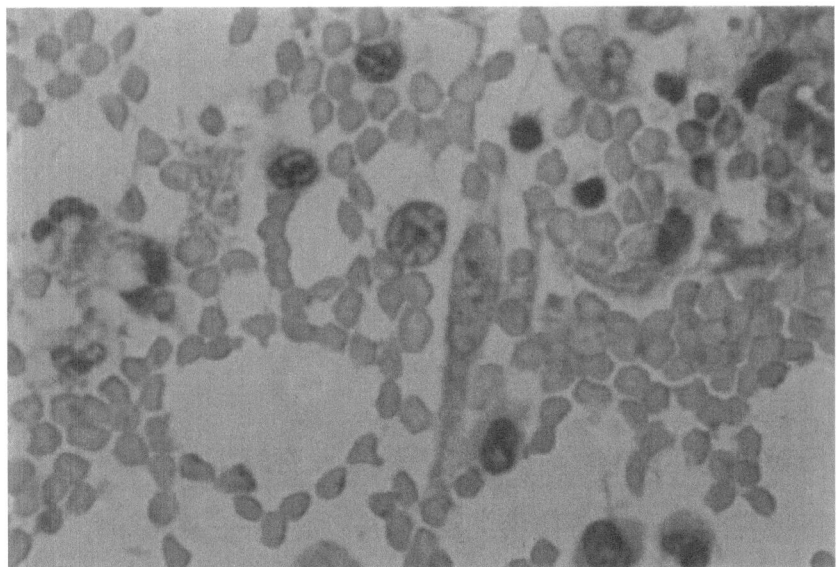

Figure 120 Mesothelioma of connective tissue type showing a single malignant stromal cell at the centre of the field. Papanicolaou stain (× 800)

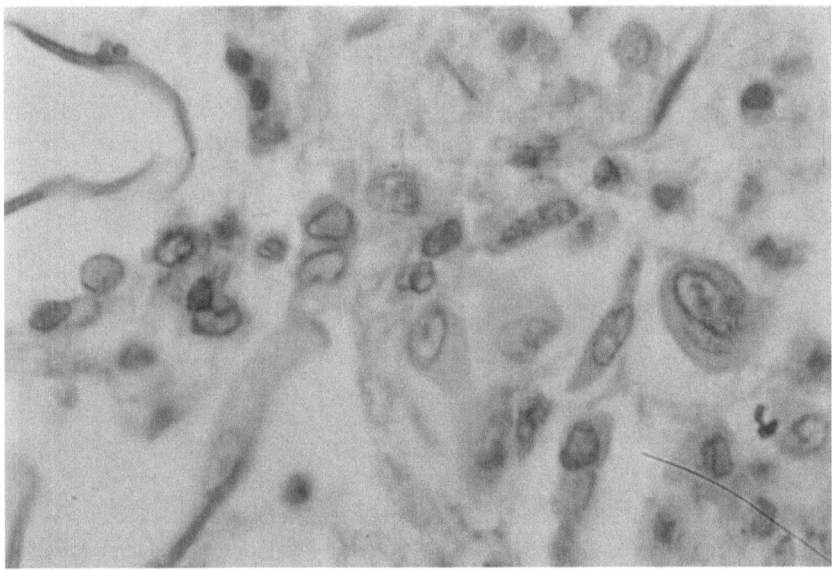

Figure 121 Section from a cell block showing a number of fibre-like cells (× 800)

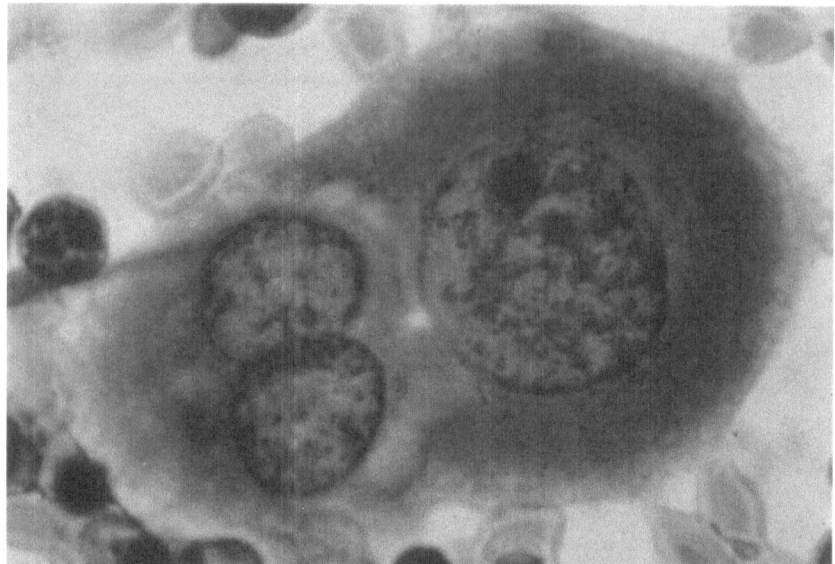

Figure 122   Two malignant mesothelioma cells at high magnification to show the irregularity of the chromatin pattern, together with the sharp angularities of the
nucleoli. The nuclear membrane appears smooth and the cytoplasm around the
nucleus is very densely stained. There is marked shading away at the periphery. The
second cell is binucleate and is much smaller. Papanicolaou stain (× 2000)

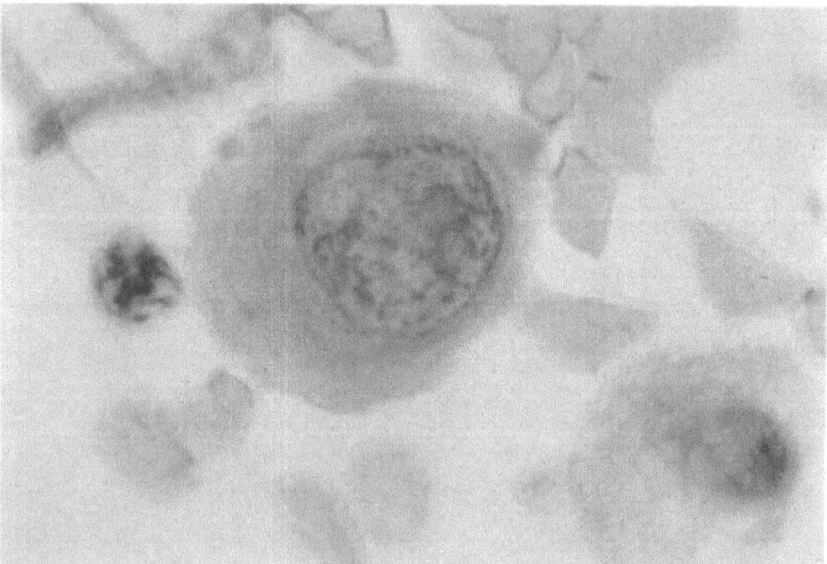

Figure 123   A single malignant mesothelial cell which shows similar features to
Figure 122 but there is some wrinkling of the nuclear membrane. Papanicolaou
stain (× 2000)

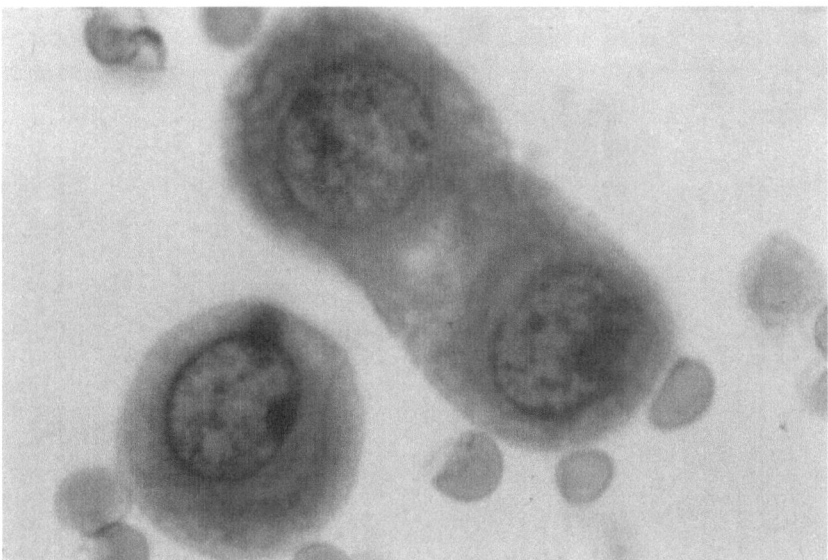

Figure 124   Contrast the three reactive mesothelial cells in this field with the previous two illustrations. The cells are smaller, and the nuclear chromatin is finely granular and regular. The nucleoli have a smooth outline. The cytoplasmic staining is slightly less dense. Papanicolaou stain (× 2000)

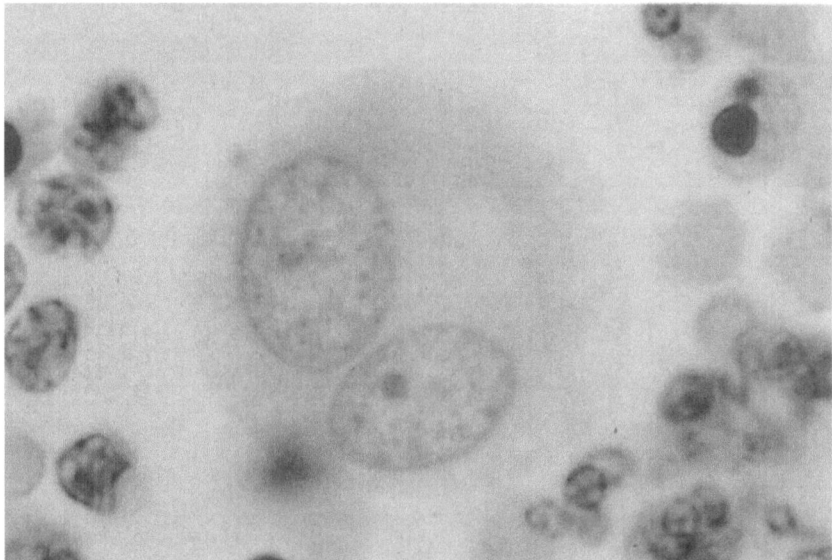

Figure 125   A larger reactive mesothelial cell which is binucleate. There is a dispersed fine granular chromatin pattern and a prominent, but uniform and smooth nucleolus in each nucleus. The cytoplasmic staining is much less dense than in malignant cells. Papanicolaou stain (× 2000)

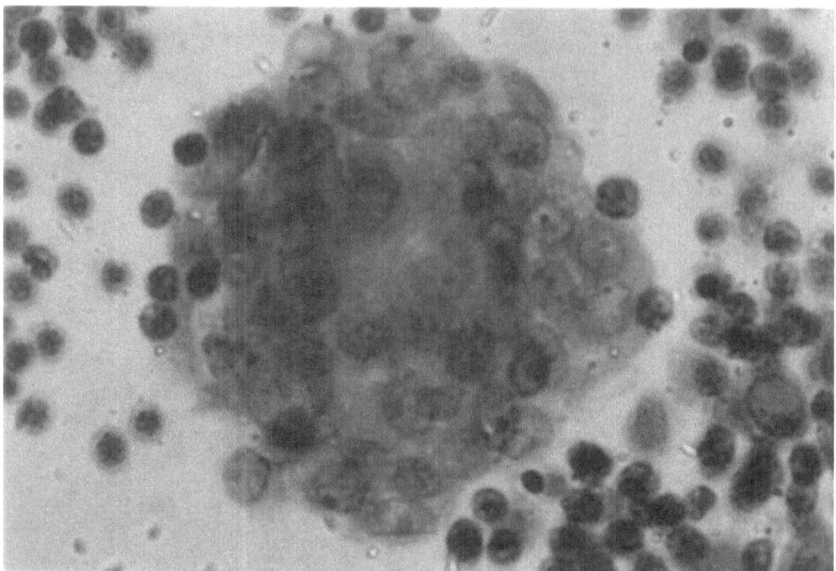

Figure 126 Compare this reactive 'raspberry-like' group with the malignant fragment in Figure 109. The nuclear chromatin pattern of the constituent cells is paler staining and at high magnification could be seen to be finely granular and regular. Papanicolaou stain (× 800)

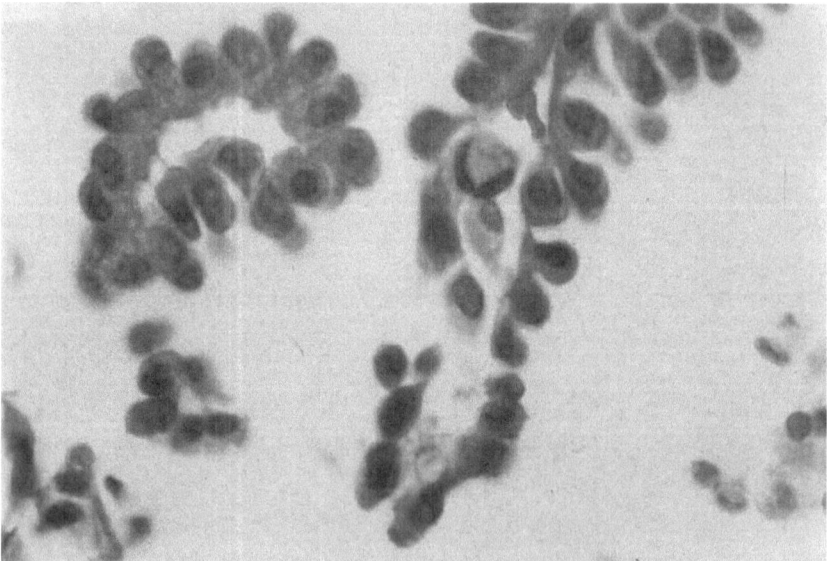

Figure 127 A tissue section from the paraffin block of a cell deposit taken from a similar case to the above in which it is much easier to recognize chains of benign mesothelial cells (× 800)

IX. CASE HISTORIES

Case No. 1
Diffuse malignant mesothelioma of the pleura – mixed type

Clinical history

A 66-year-old man. In 1969 he had an isolated episode of pleurisy. In 1977 he complained of dyspnoea, weakness, loss of weight. He was found to have a left-sided pleural effusion. No malignant tumour cells were found in the pleural fluid.

In October, 1978 an exploratory thoracotomy revealed a fleshy infiltration of the left pleura and pericardium, several centimetres thick. The biopsy appearances are shown in the illustrations that follow. Post-operative irradiation was given.

The patient died in September 1979.

Occupational history

The patient had been a mechanic.

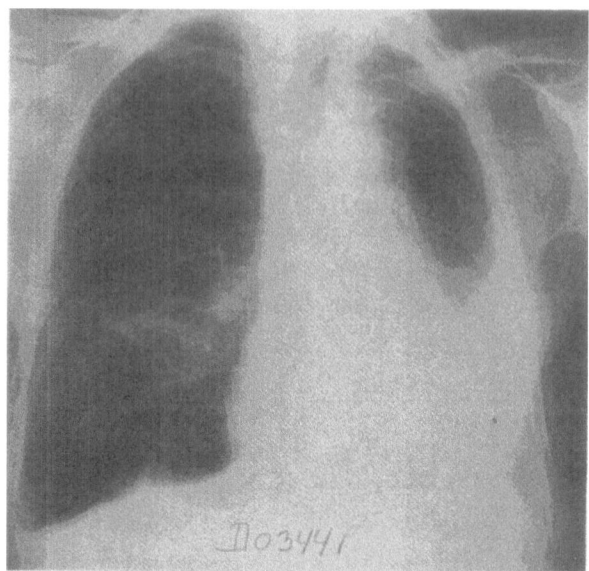

Figure 128 P.A. view of chest to show pleural thickening on the right side.
Shadowing involving the left lower zone and generalized thickening of the pleura

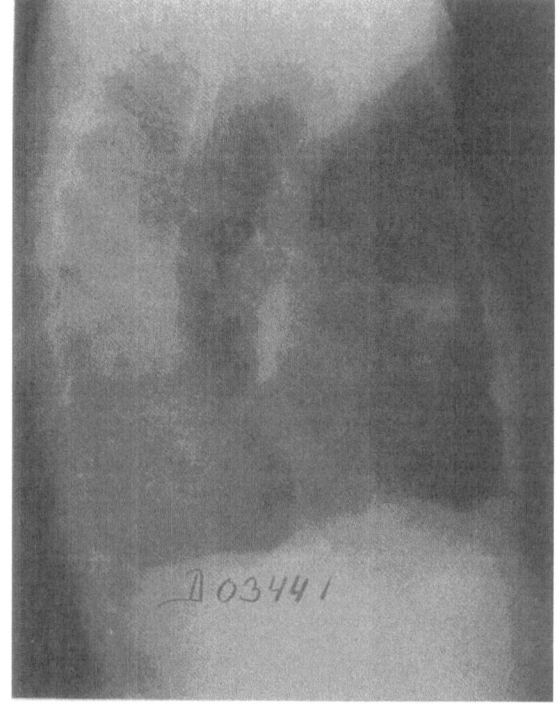

Figure 129 Lateral
view of chest showing
pleural effusion and
thickening

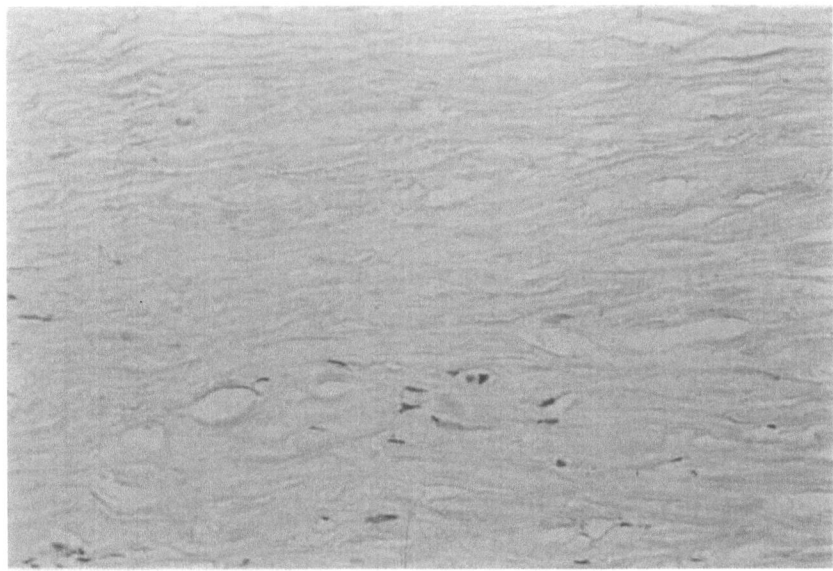

Figure 130 Thoracotomy specimen of a pleural plaque showing classical 'basket weave' appearance (× 275)

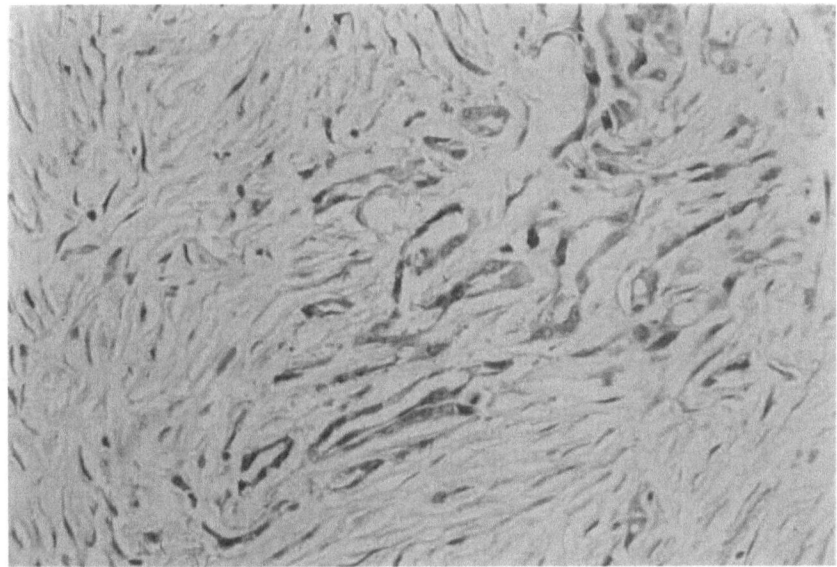

Figure 131 Thoracotomy specimen of pleural tumour. Multiple clefts and tubules lined by cuboidal and flattened cells representing the epithelial component; connective tissue components are more prominent in the periphery (× 275)

CASE HISTORIES

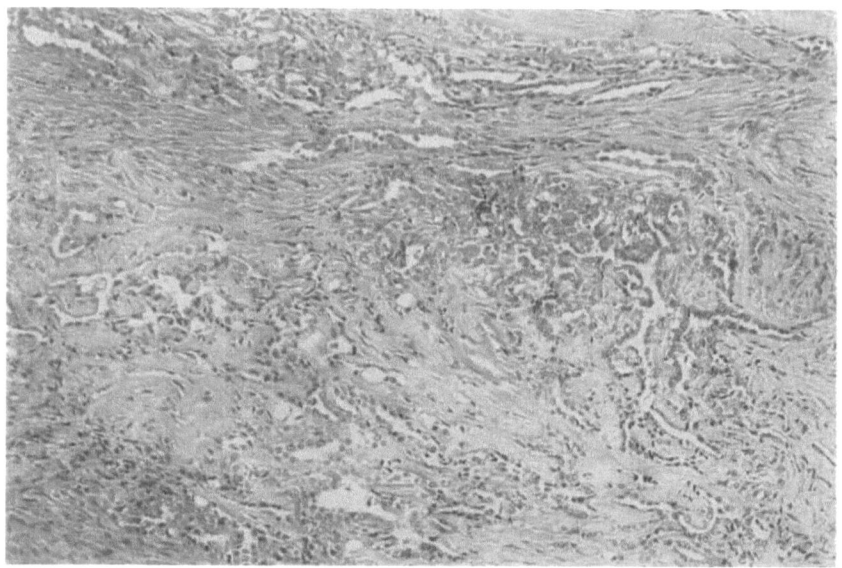

Figure 132 Epithelial and connective tissue components of a mesothelioma (× 110)

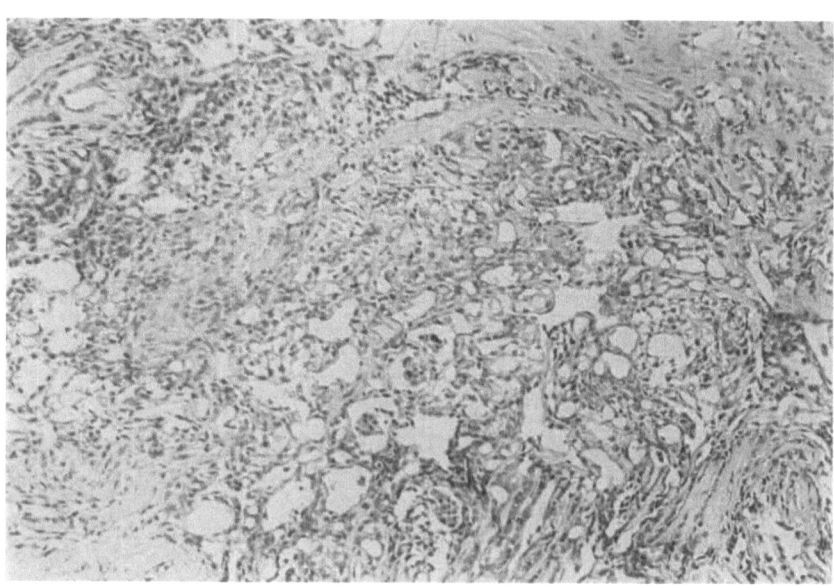

Figure 133 Epithelial and connective tissue components of a mesothelioma (× 110)

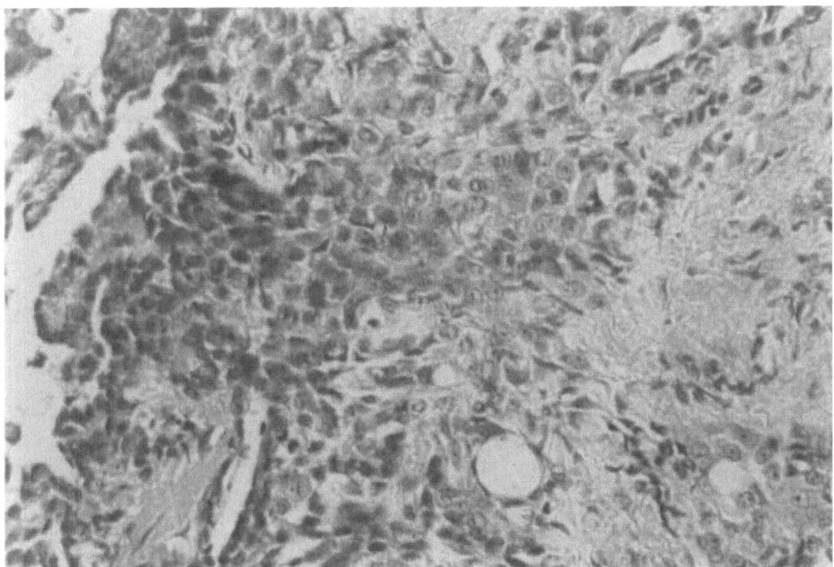

Figure 134   Surface of the tumour showing papillary and solid epithelial elements (× 275)

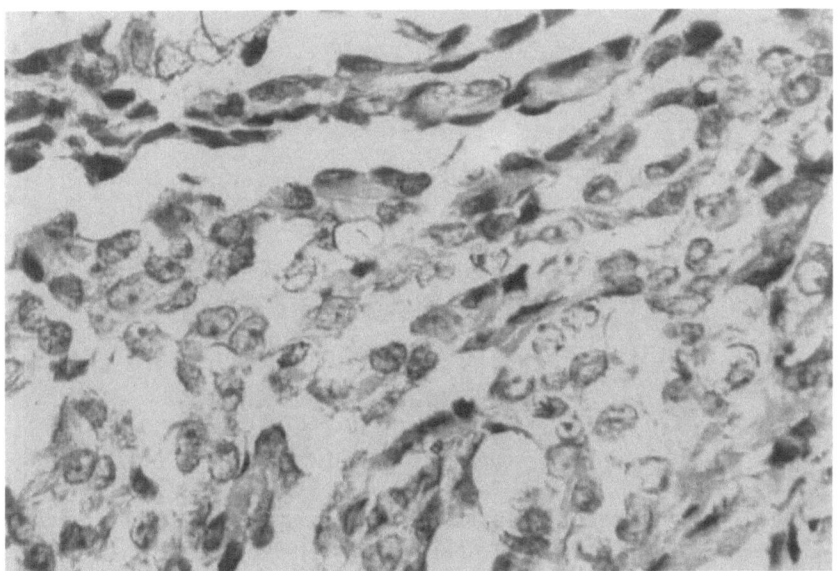

Figure 135   High power view showing cellular detail of epithelial type cells (× 730)

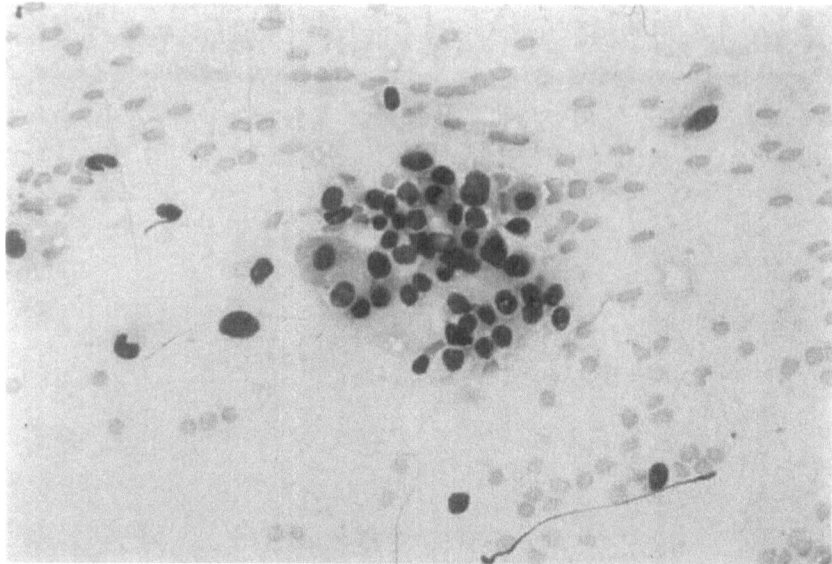

Figure 136 Cytology smears prepared from imprints showing large and small cell types. May-Grünwald–Giemsa stain (× 275)

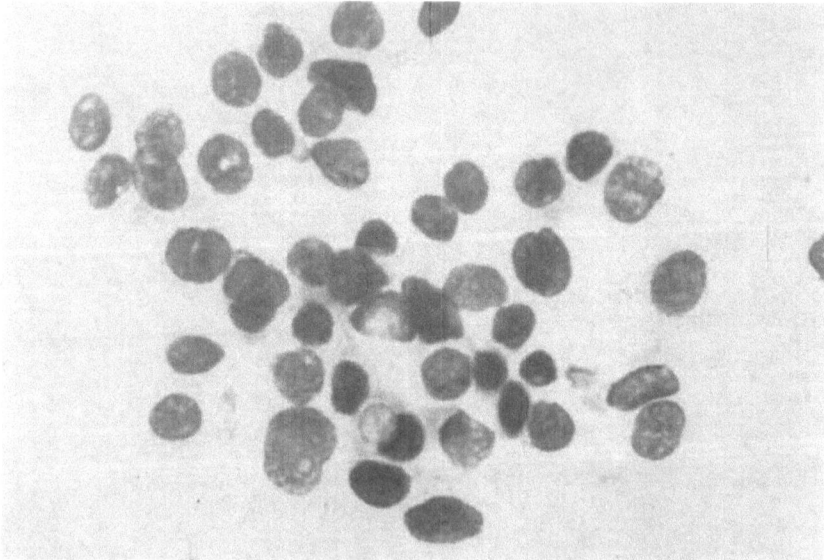

Figure 137 Higher magnification showing epithelial type cells with abundant pale cytoplasm and large irregular nuclei with a coarse chromatin structure. In between, smaller and darker cells, poor in cytoplasm, are present. May-Grünwald–Giemsa stain (× 800)

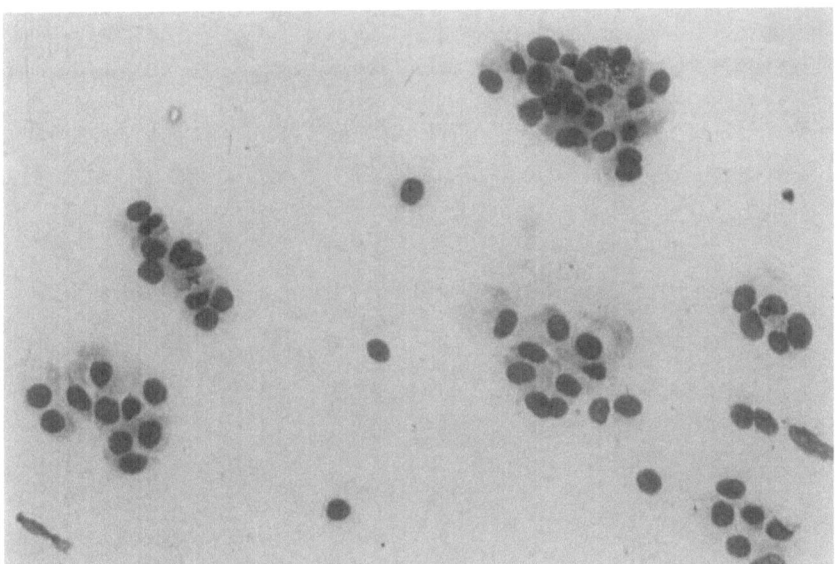

Figure 138 Scattered clusters of epithelial-like cells. May-Grünwald–Giemsa stain (× 275)

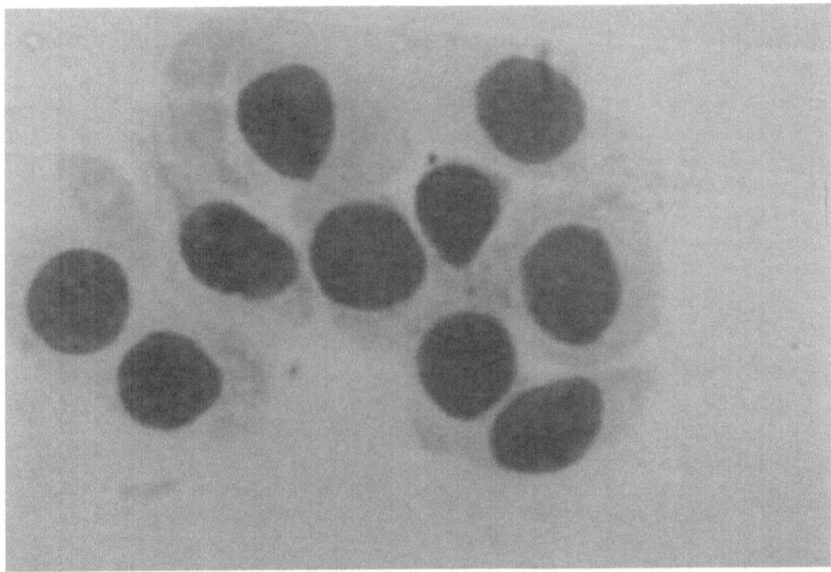

Figure 139 Higher magnification of a cluster to demonstrate the paucity of nucleoli (in contrast to the appearance of carcinoma cells). May-Grünwald–Giemsa stain (× 1350)

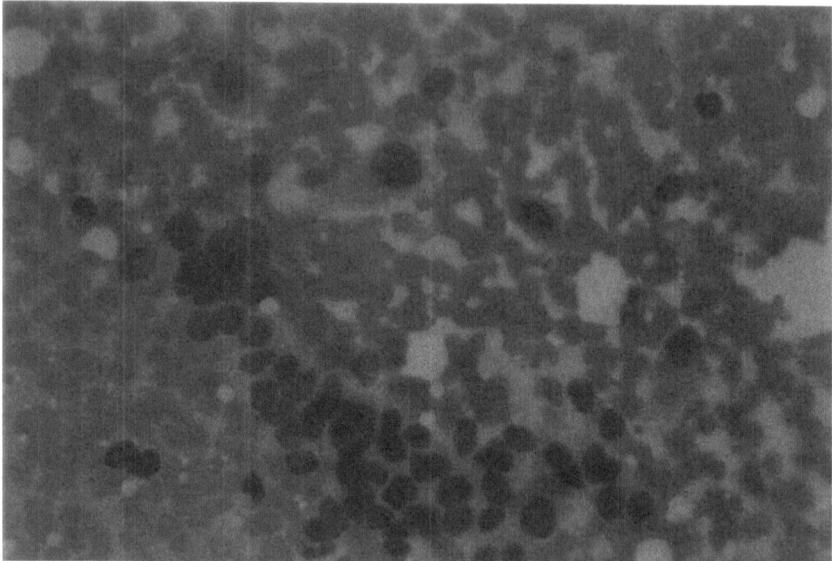

Figure 140 A cluster of small cells and scattered, single large epithelial-like cells. May-Grünwald–Giemsa stain (× 430)

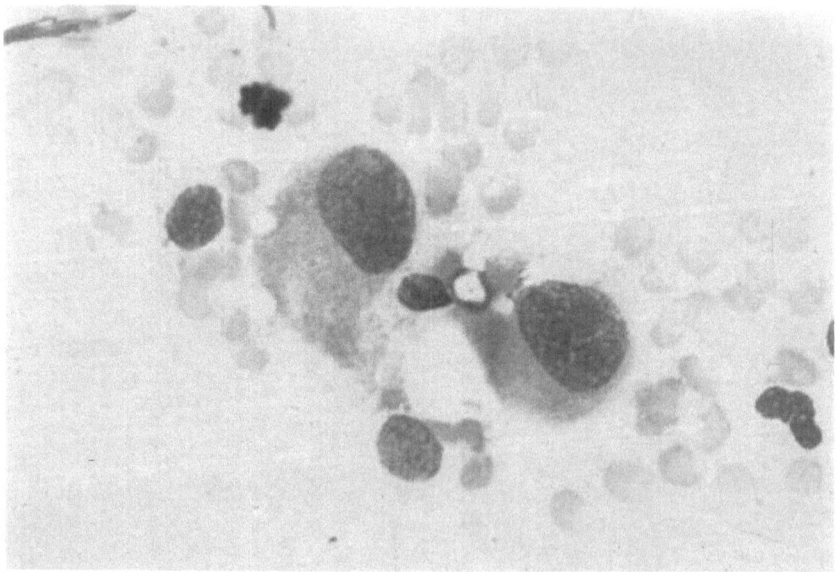

Figure 141 High power view of two large epithelial-like cells with several ill-defined nucleoli, more in keeping with mesothelioma than carcinoma. Two small cells with similar nuclear structure are also present. May-Grünwald–Giemsa stain (× 800)

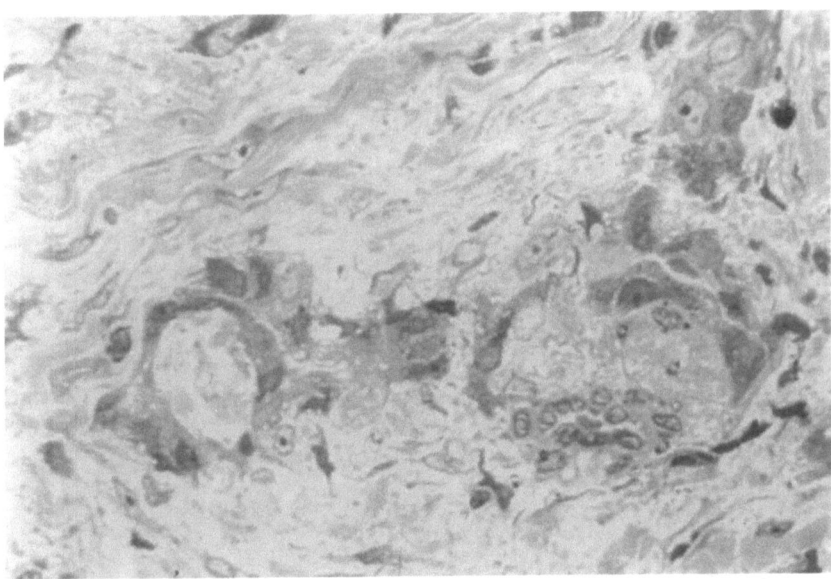

Figure 142 1 μm thick toluidine blue stain showing rounded epithelial elements. In the top left corner two elongated connective tissue type cells are seen (× 730)

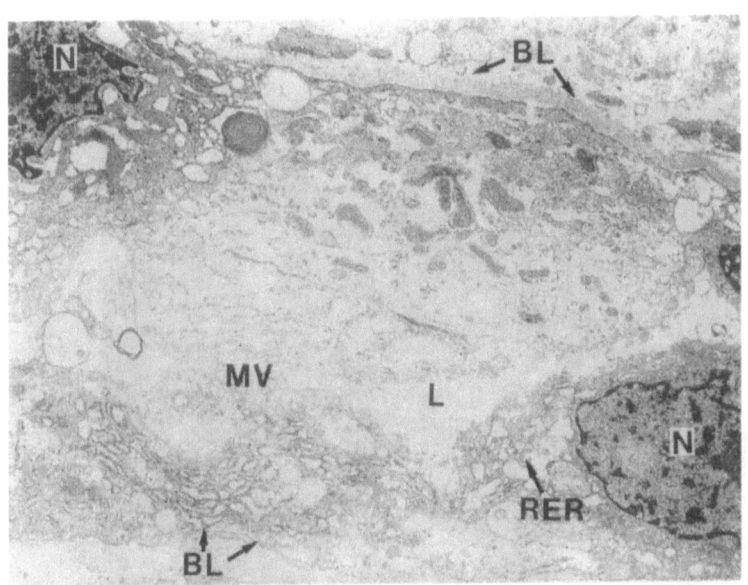

Figure 143 Electron microscopy (EM)* shows the characteristic ultrastructural features of a mesothelioma. These are (1) large irregular indented nucleus (bottom right edge), (2) intra-cytoplasmic microfilaments with a diameter of 70–100 Å, (3) numerous long and slender microvilli, (4) thickened basal lamina (× 5000)

*Key for electronmicroscopy follows Figure 145

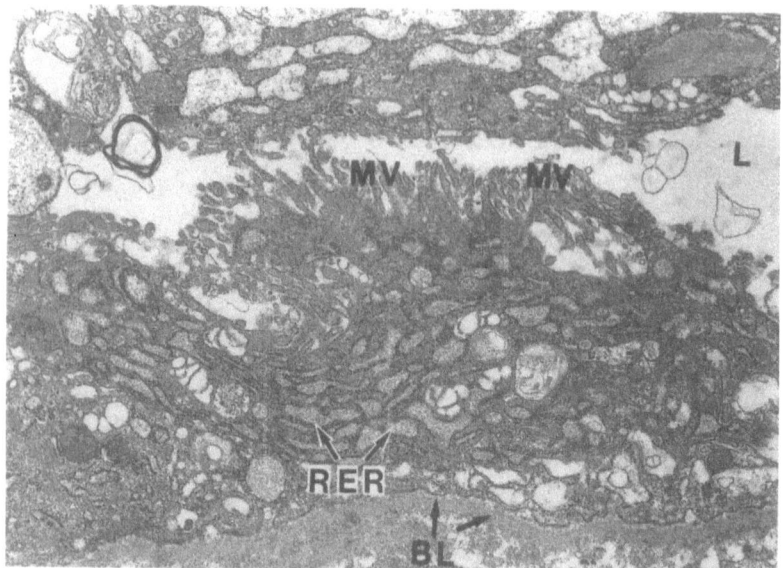

Figure 144   EM shows the microvilli at a higher magnification (× 10 000)

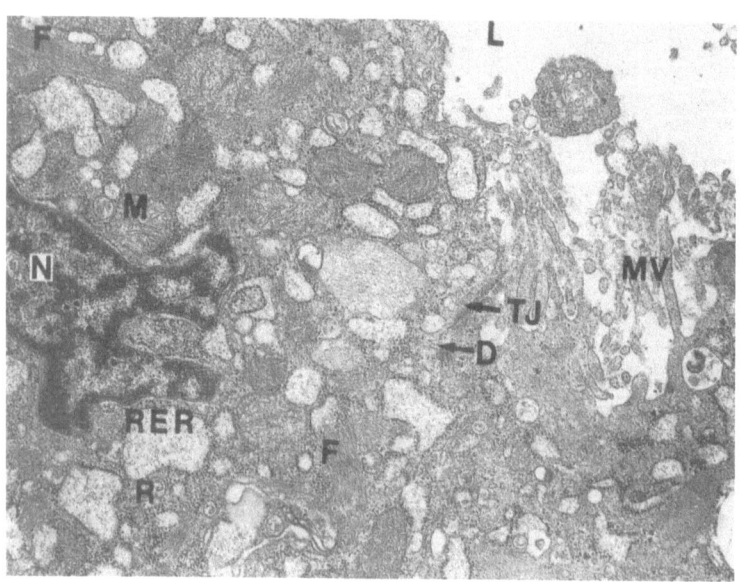

Figure 145   EM shows the abnormal indented nucleus and the different intracytoplasmic organelles, tight junctions and desmosomes (× 12 500)

Key for electron microscope (EM) figures:

B.L.	Basal lamina
M.V.	Microvilli
L	Lumen
R.E.R.	Rough endoplasmic reticulum
M	Mitochondria
R	Ribosomes
F	Intra-cytoplasmic microfilaments
D	Desmosomes
T.J.	Tight junction

Acknowledgement

The authors are grateful to Dr Stein Paulsen for the electron microscopy investigation and interpretation of this case.

Case No. 2
Diffuse malignant mesothelioma of the peritoneum – mixed type

Clinical history

A 56-year-old man. In March 1965 he had general complaints thought to be due to flu. Chest x-ray was normal. Asbestos bodies were detected in the sputum. In June 1965 he developed symptoms due to mild lead intoxication. He resumed work, but was later re-admitted to hospital in August 1965 with vague abdominal pain and ascites. Cytological examination of the ascitic fluid was suggestive of mesothelioma. A laparotomy revealed several serosal tumour deposits and a metastasis in the liver. No primary tumour was found. The histological appearance of the biopsy was thought to be either a metastasis from a carcinoma or a mesothelioma. Chemotherapy was given but the patient gradually deteriorated and he died in May 1966.

Occupational history

1930–40 he had been a cook's mate on a ship.
From 1940–5 he had a variety of jobs.
From 1945–6 he worked at a shipyard, firstly as a rust scraper and subsequently as a painter.

Autopsy findings

2 litres of ascitic fluid were present. The peritoneum was diffusely covered with a tumour mass which did not penetrate deeply into the underlying tissue. The right parietal pleura showed scattered tumour nodules. No other metastases were present. No other primary tumour was found.

Microscopy showed diffuse malignant mesothelioma of mixed type. The presence of foci of necrosis may have been influenced by the chemotherapy. The difference in appearance between the biopsy and the autopsy histology could be due to sampling, to the progression of malignancy in the time interval or to the chemotherapy.

The lung tissue contained many asbestos bodies.

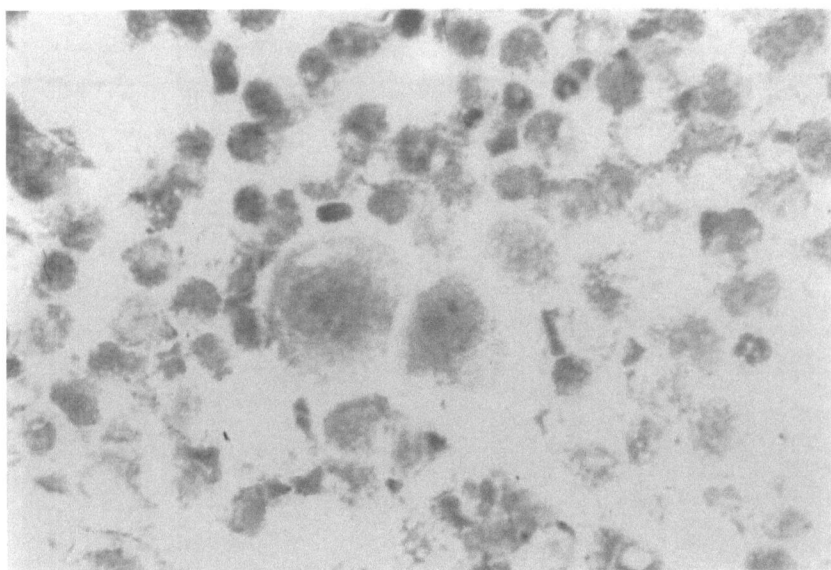

Figure 146 Cytology of ascitic fluid shows cellular-rich fluid, with considerable pleomorphism. Two large epithelial-like cells are present in the centre. One of these is multinucleated. May-Grünwald–Giemsa stain (× 730)

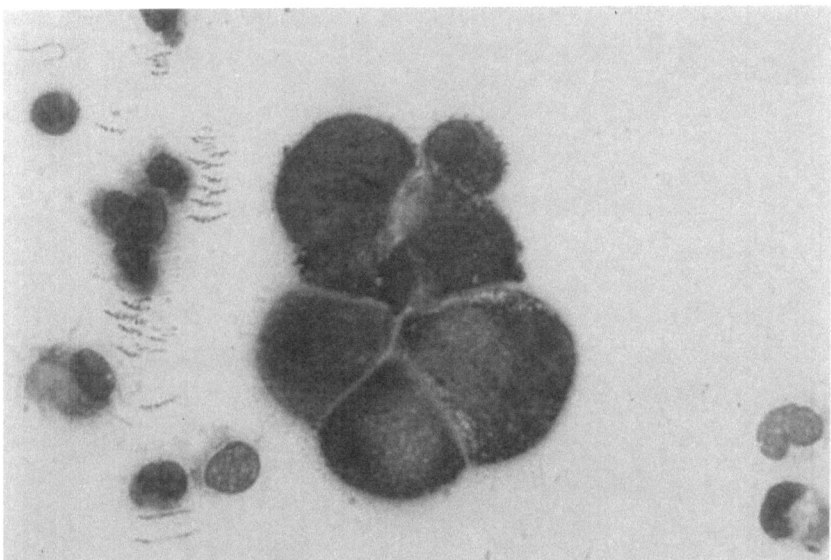

Figure 147 A cluster of malignant cells with eccentrically-placed nuclei, multiple ill-defined nucleoli and coarse chromatin structure. There is marked anisocytosis and pleomorphism. The cytoplasm shows variation in its staining property. May-Grünwald–Giemsa stain (× 730)

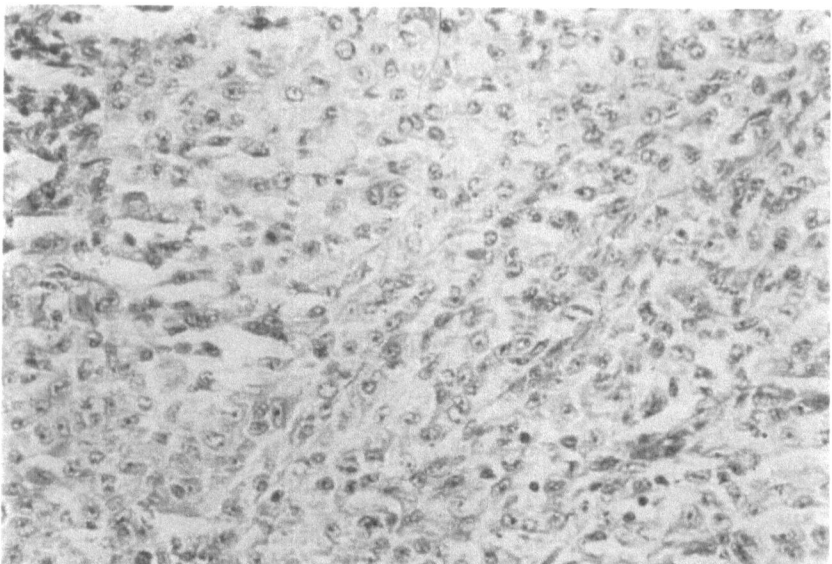

Figure 148 Biopsy specimen taken 10 days after cytological examination shows a predominantly epithelial type tumour ($\times$ 275)

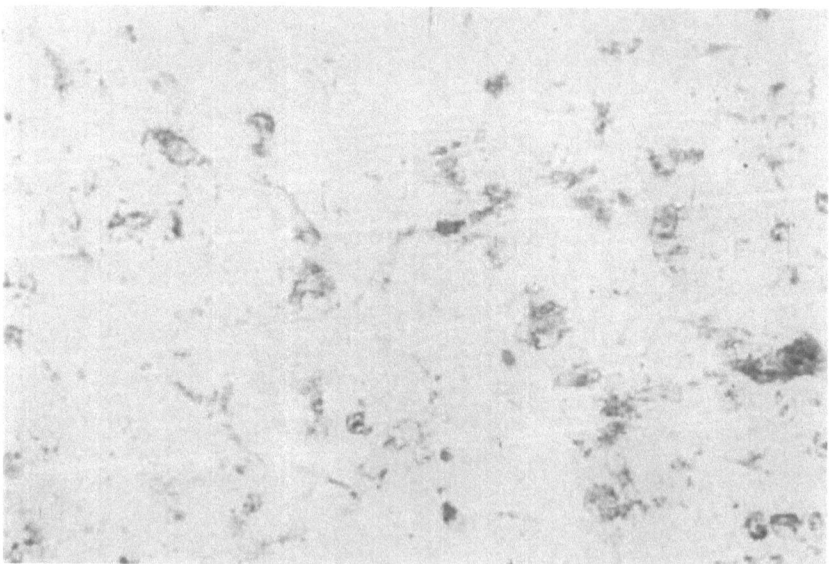

Figure 149 A high power view of the tumour shows no intracellular mucin. The only positively stained material is in intercellular substance. At this stage the biopsy appearance cannot differentiate with certainty between a mesothelioma and a carcinoma. PAS stain ($\times$ 730)

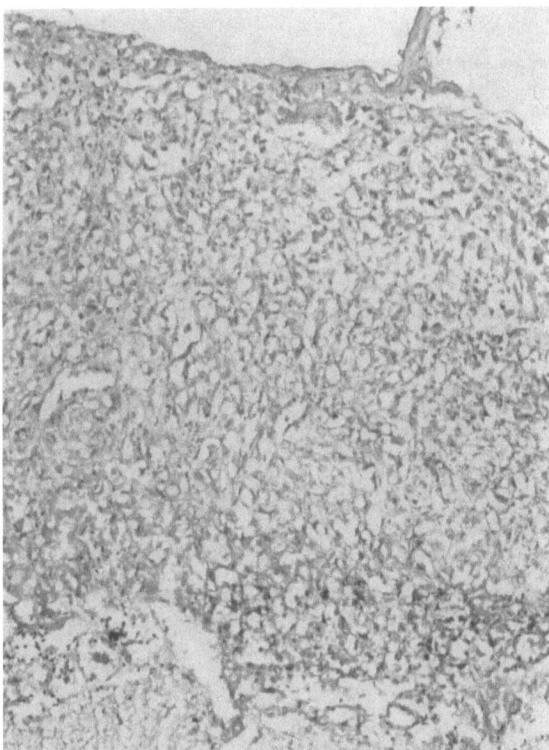

Figure 150 Autopsy specimen of tumour on the outer surface of the intestinal wall. In this section there is a fairly sharp demarcation between the tumour and the muscular layer of the intestine ($\times$ 110)

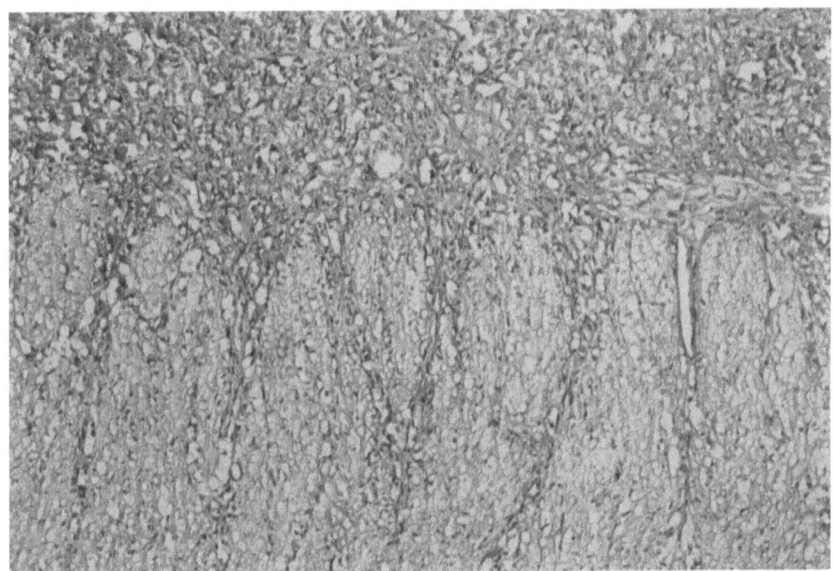

Figure 151 In other sites there is spiky but shallow invasion of the outer muscle layer by the tumour ($\times$ 110)

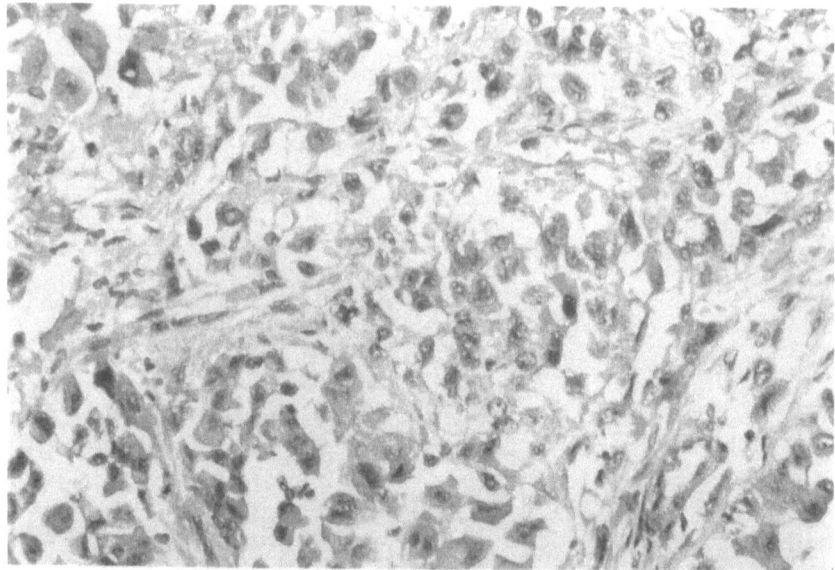

Figure 152 The tumour is a mixed type mesothelioma of rather poorly differentiated appearance. There is scattered individual cell necrosis (× 275)

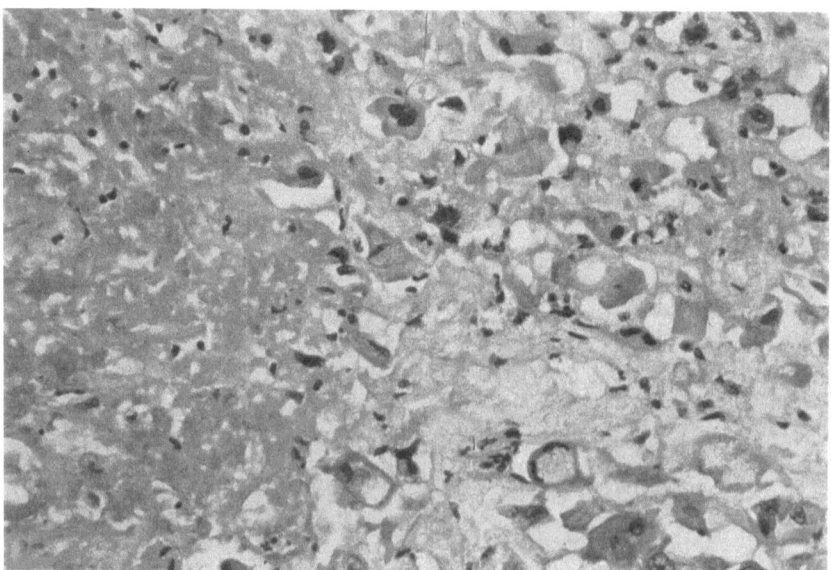

Figure 153 Parts of the tumour show foci of necrosis with surrounding pleomorphic cells and giant cells (× 275)

Case No. 3
Diffuse malignant mesothelioma of the pleura – connective tissue type

Clinical history

A 62-year-old man. In April 1979 he was admitted to hospital with a left-sided pleural effusion. 2 litres of fluid were removed. Cytology of the clot was suspicious of mesothelioma cells. X-ray of the chest six weeks after admission revealed nodular tumour masses in the left thoracic cavity.

No treatment was given.

The patient died in May 1979.

Occupational history

The patient was a farm labourer and later a sawmill labourer. No known history of asbestos exposure was elicited.

Autopsy findings

The left pleura showed diffuse and nodular fleshy tumour, forming adhesions and loculated areas. No metastases were found and no primary tumour in any other organ was detected.

Microscopy of many of the sections showed an exclusively connective tissue type of tumour. More pleomorphic cells were seen in later sections, and after further sampling (Figures 169 and beyond) the presence of epithelial-like areas became apparent.

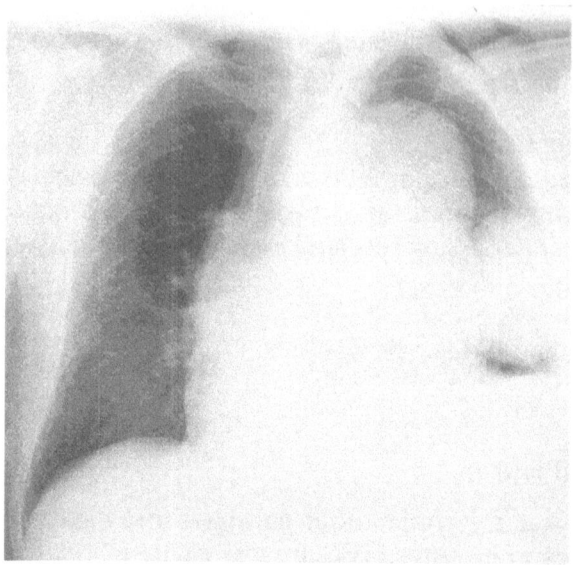

Figure 154   P.A. view of chest shows nodular shadowing
and effusion in the left thoracic cavity

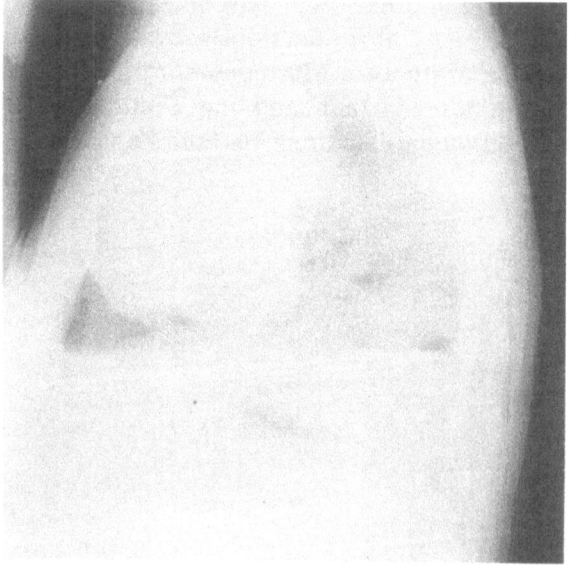

Figure 155   Lateral view of above

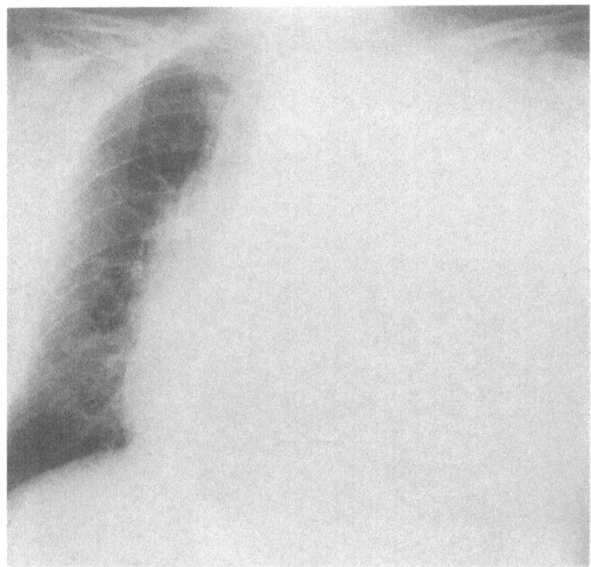

Figure 156 P.A. view of chest six weeks after previous X-ray to show total opacity of left thoracic cavity

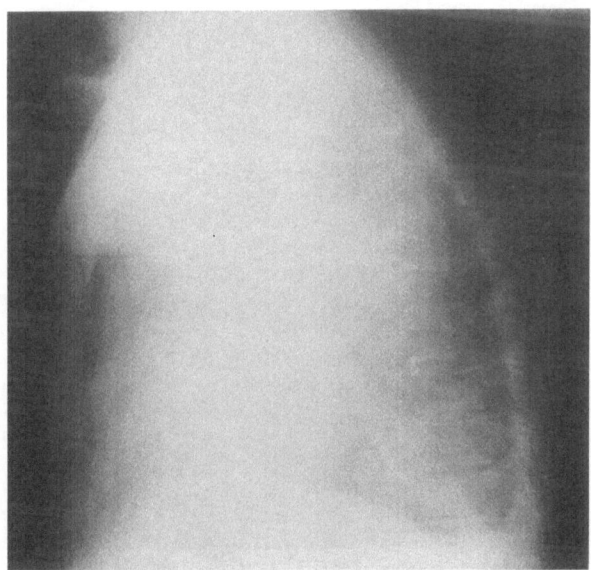

Figure 157 Lateral view of above showing that the opacity is due to tumour and not to effusion

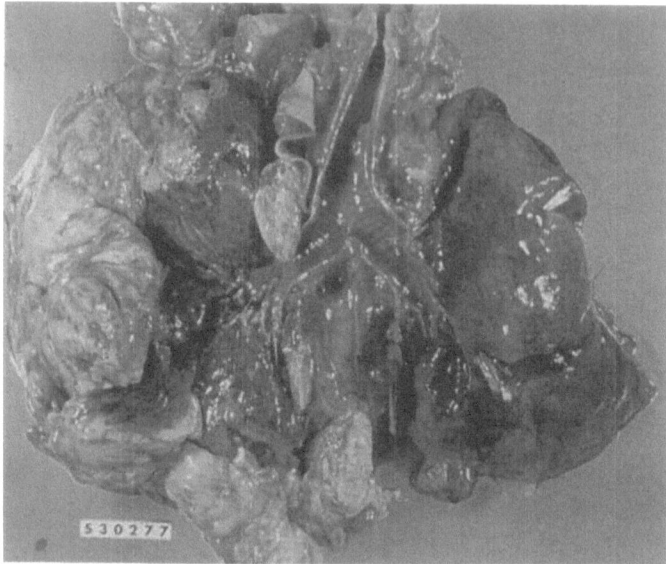

Figure 158 Autopsy specimen shows diffuse tumour of the left pleura with partly nodular appearance

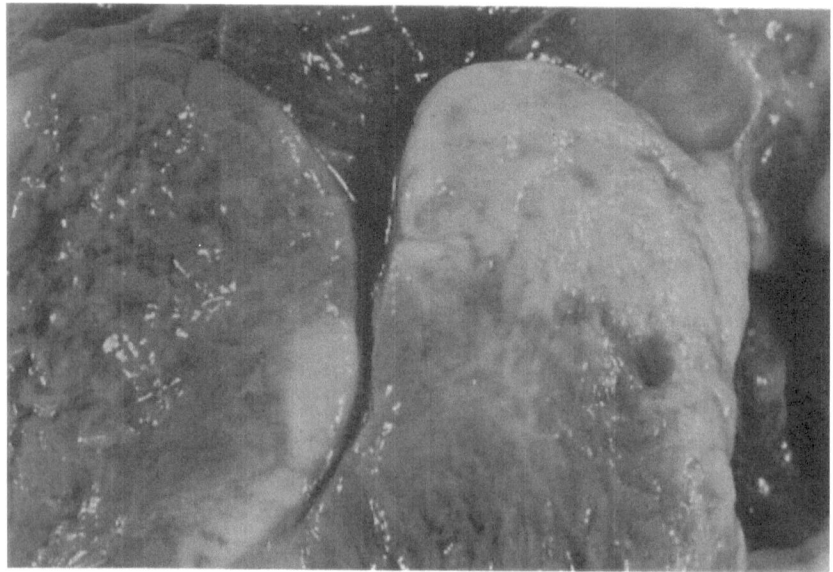

Figure 159 A close-up view of the cut surface of the above tumour. It has a fleshy sarcoma-like appearance and a nodular, sharp demarcation at the junction of the lung parenchyma

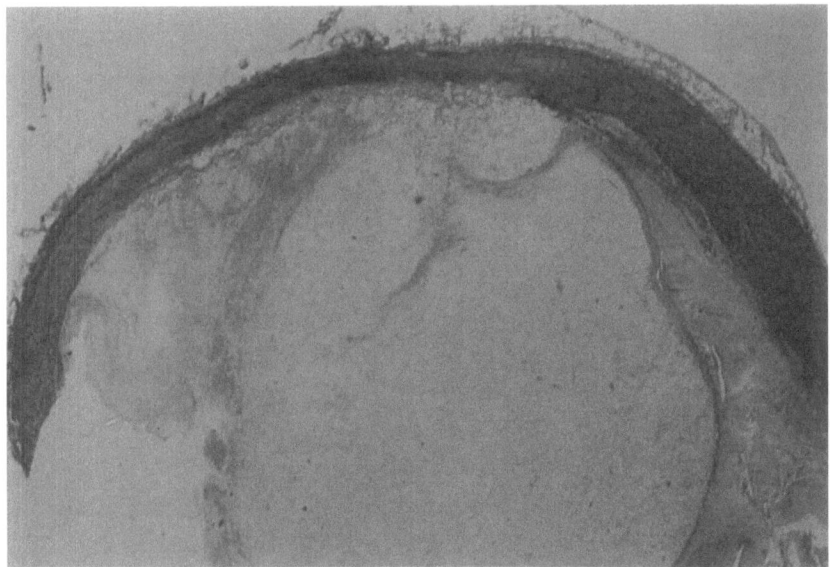

Figure 160   Low power view of tumour within the pulmonary artery. Van Gieson
elastic stain ($\times$ 6.5)

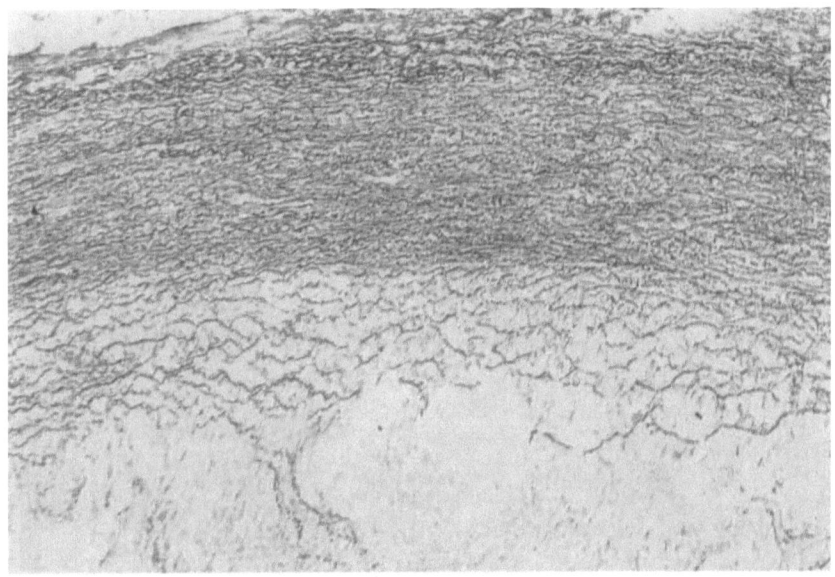

Figure 161   A higher magnification of the above showing partial destruction of the
inner vessel wall. Van Gieson elastic stain ($\times$ 45)

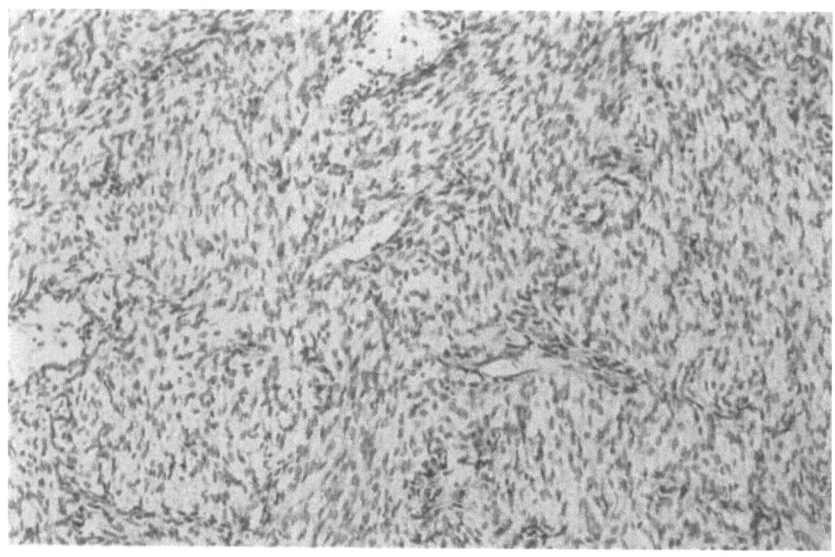

Figure 162 A cellular rich area of connective tissue type. Several thin-walled blood vessels are present ($\times$ 110)

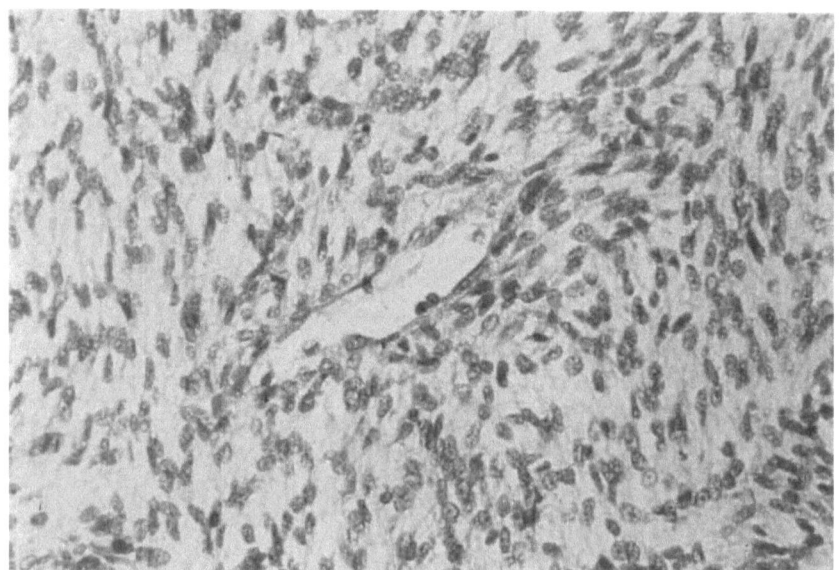

Figure 163 Higher magnification of above, showing a whorled pattern of spindle cells, cut in diverse planes with a blood vessel at the centre ($\times$ 275)

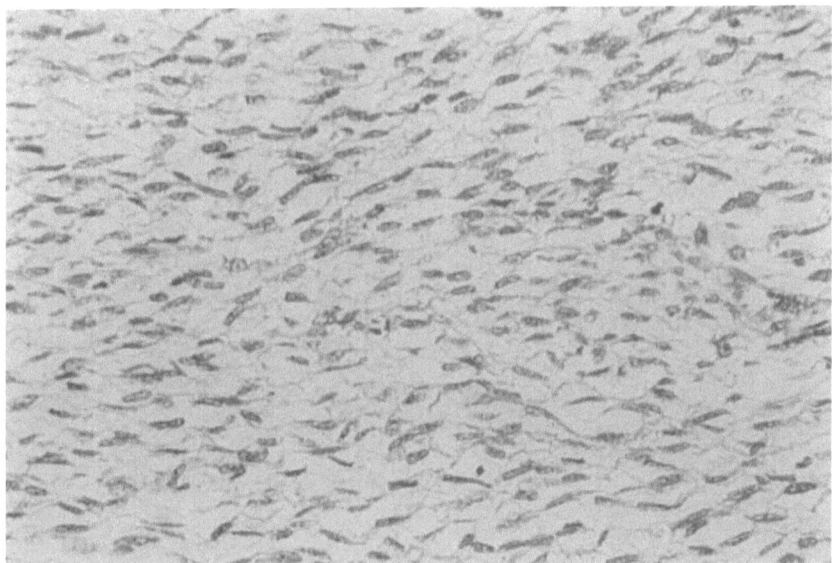

Figure 164 Further view of the same tumour showing spindle cells in a wavy pattern (× 275)

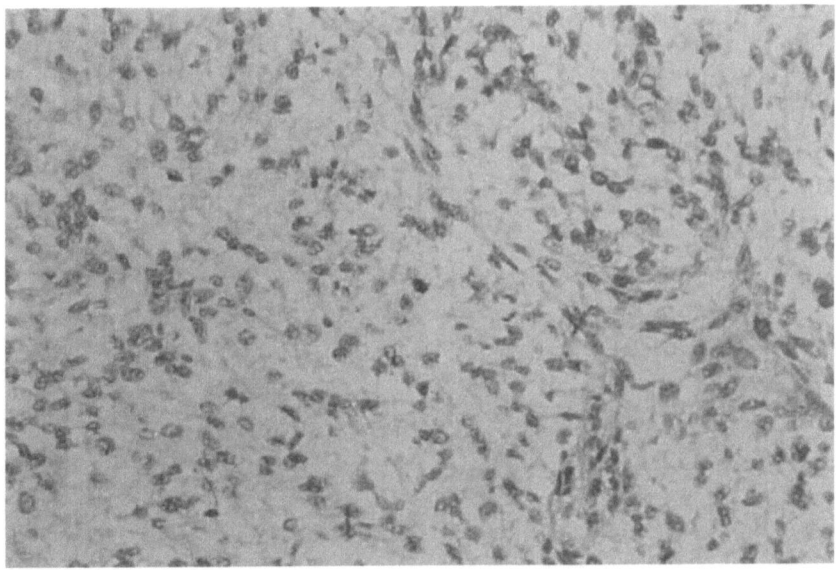

Figure 165 A mixture of elongated spindle cells and more blunted cells in an irregular arrangement. (× 275)

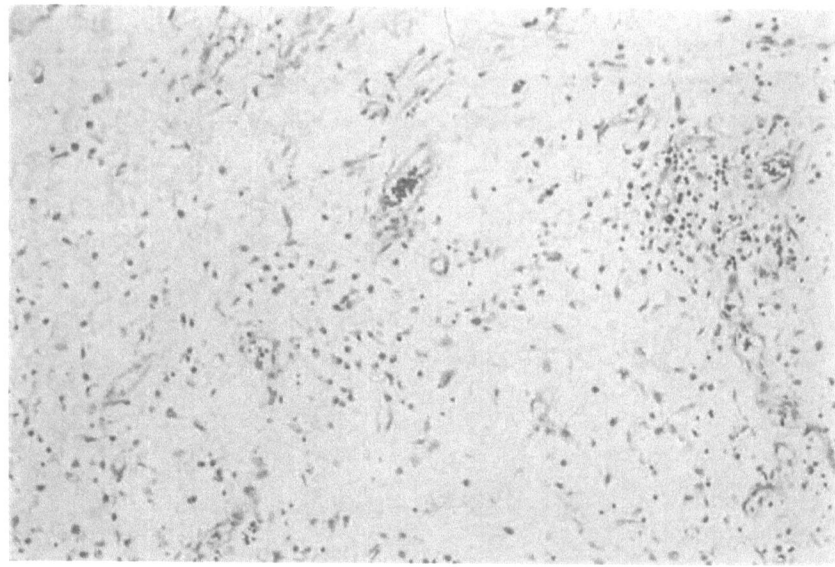

Figure 166 A further view of the same tumour shows less cellularity (× 110)

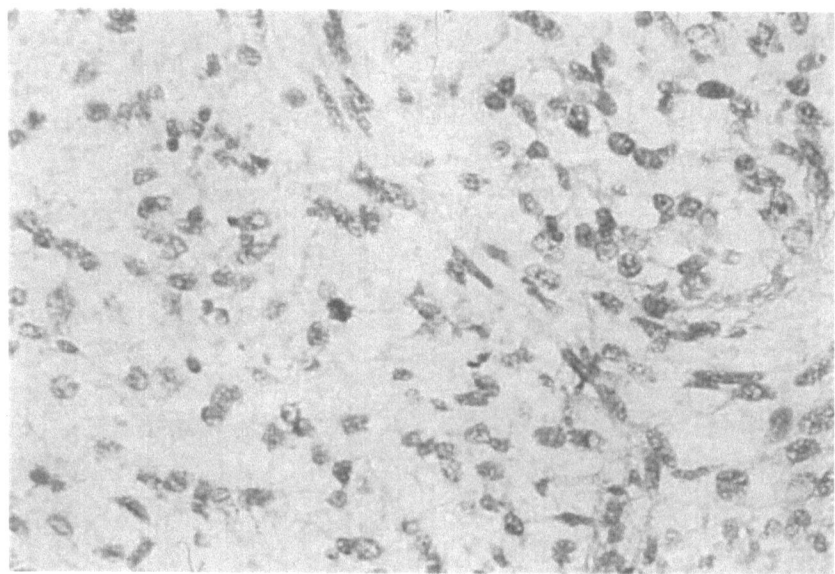

Figure 167 Higher power view of Figure 165. There is a gradual transition from spindle cells to the more blunted cells. A single mitosis is seen at the centre (× 430)

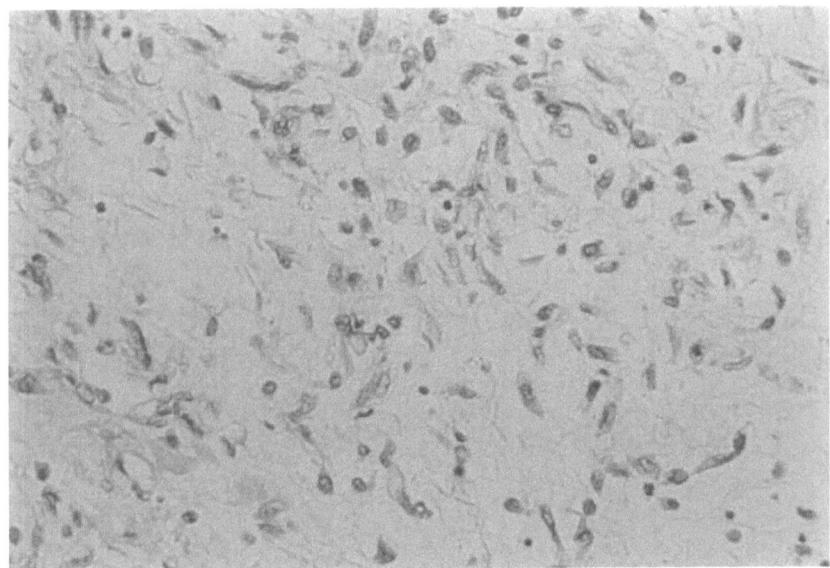

Figure 168 An area dominated by more myxoid, loosely arranged stroma. The cells are slightly more pleomorphic than those seen previously (× 275)

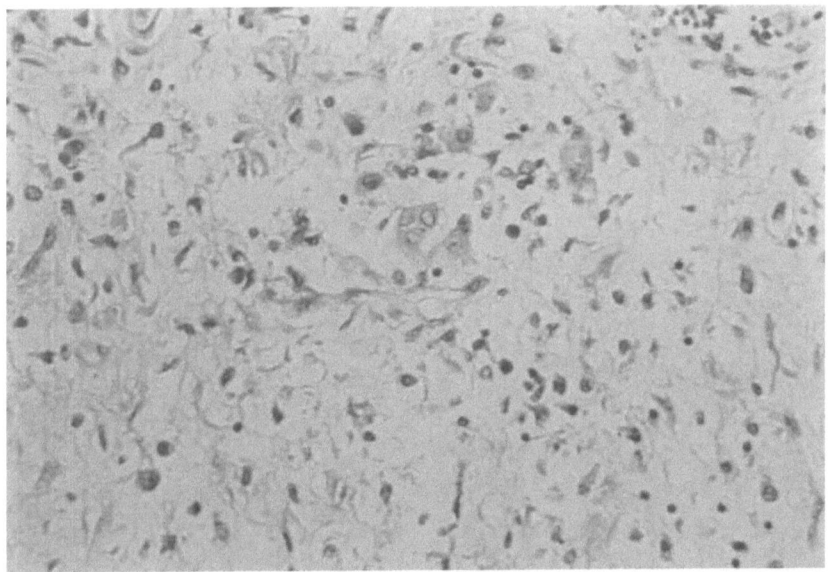

Figure 169 Same magnification as above. The stroma is similar, but at the centre a small group of cells is present with a more epithelial type differentiation. Scattered lymphocytes and plasma cells are also present (× 275)

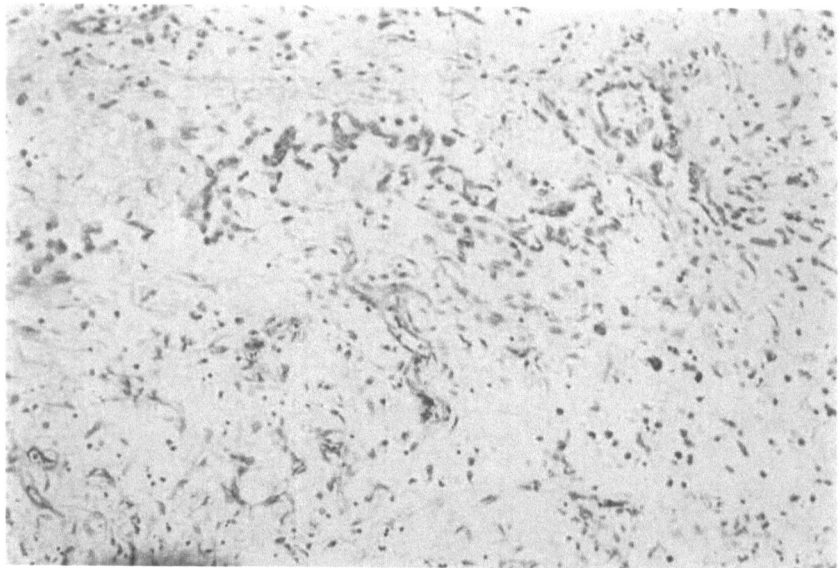

Figure 170 Low power view of another area which shows tubules and clefts, lined by a single layer of cuboidal cells (× 110)

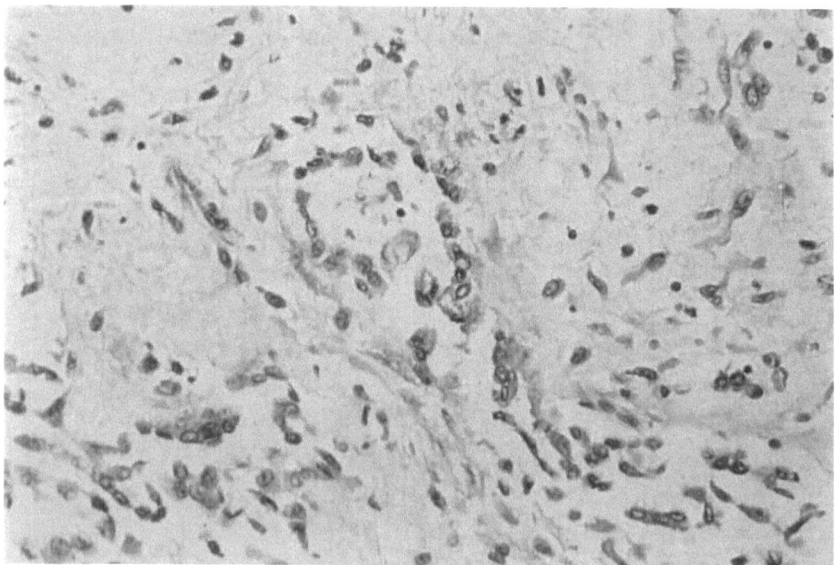

Figure 171 A higher power view of the above, showing the gradual transition between connective tissue and epithelial elements (× 275)

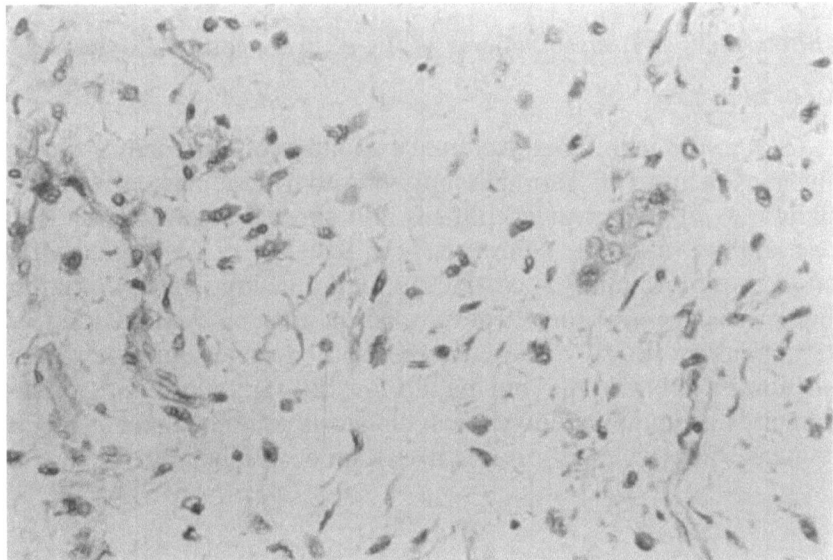

Figure 172 Another area shows similar features to those seen in Figures 170 and 171 (× 275)

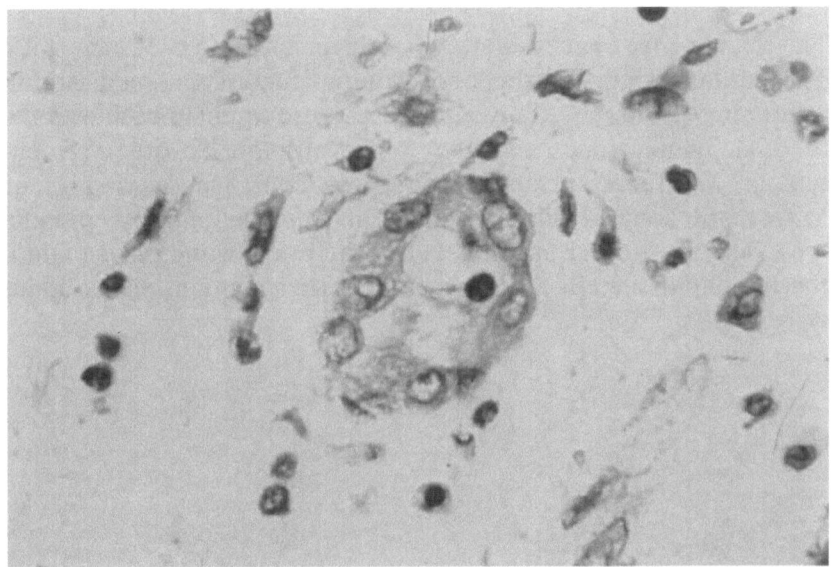

Figure 173 A higher power view of the epithelial type component (× 730)

Case No. 4
Diffuse malignant mesothelioma of the pleura – epithelial type

Clinical history

A 63-year-old man. He developed a spontaneous pneumothorax on the left side in 1973. Thoracoscopy showed hyaline thickening of the pleura. A biopsy revealed fibrosis and chronic inflammation. Talc was applied into the pleural cavity. Because of residual cavities surgical exploration was carried out and a leaking emphysematous bulla was excised. From 1974 onwards he suffered from pain in the left shoulder. In 1976 x-ray examination revealed multiple round shadows in both lungs, but mainly on the right side. No primary tumour was found and no clinical diagnosis could be made. Later in that year he developed progressive dyspnoea and died.

Occupational history

Worked in the building trade and was in contact with cement and asbestos.

Autopsy findings

The left lung was encapsulated by a layer of tumour 1–2 cm thick. The tumour infiltrated the pericardium, diaphragm, mediastinum and intercostal tissue. Many metastases were found in both lungs, in the hilar lymph nodes and in the myocardium. No other primary tumour was found in any organ. Pleural plaques were present. Microscopy showed diffuse malignant mesothelioma of epithelial type. Talc was found on the level of the pre-existing pleura and in the tumour tissue. In the lung parenchyma many asbestos bodies were present.

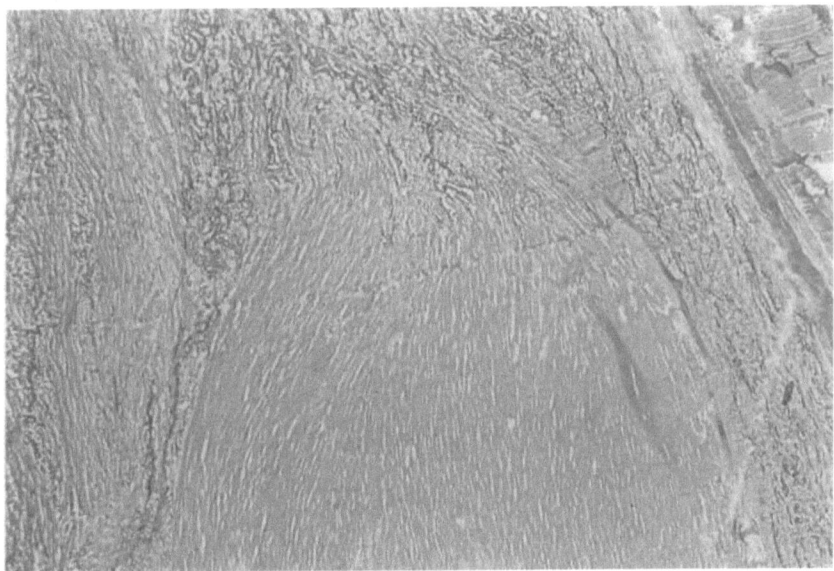

Figure 174 Low power view of a pleural plaque with tumour on both sides, and also invading the plaque (× 45)

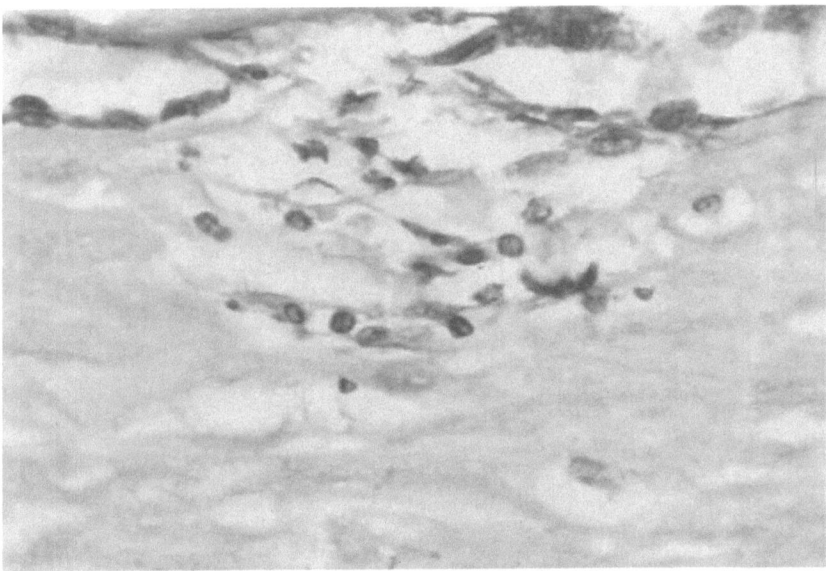

Figure 175 High power view of border zone between the tumour and the plaque (× 730)

Figure 176   The mesothelioma is of mainly epithelial type ($\times$ 275)

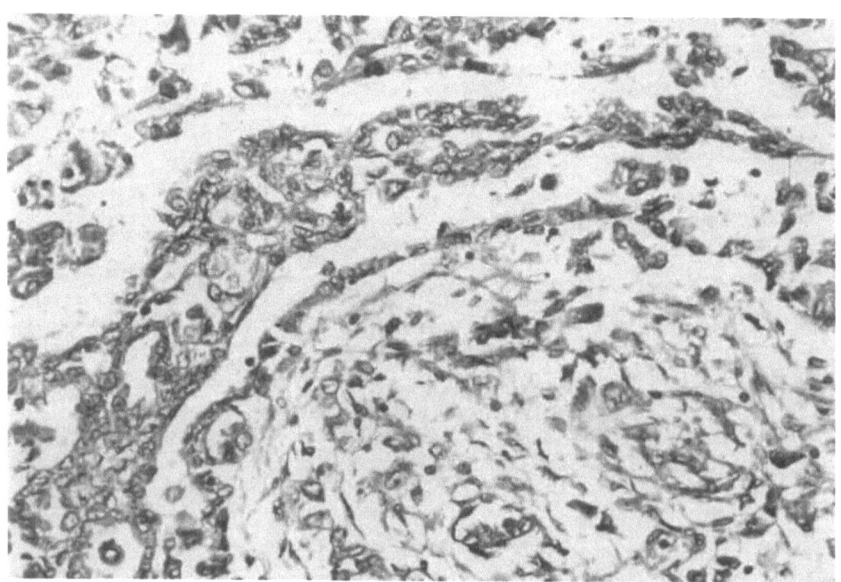

Figure 177   Both epithelial and connective tissue components are present ($\times$ 275)

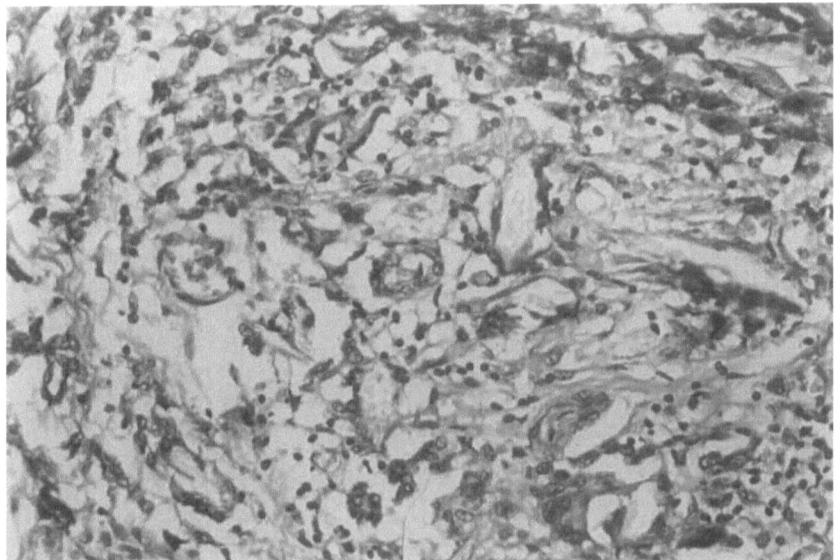

Figure 178 Slight lymphocytic infiltration and foreign body reaction within the tumour are obscuring the degree of differentiation of tumour in this field (× 275)

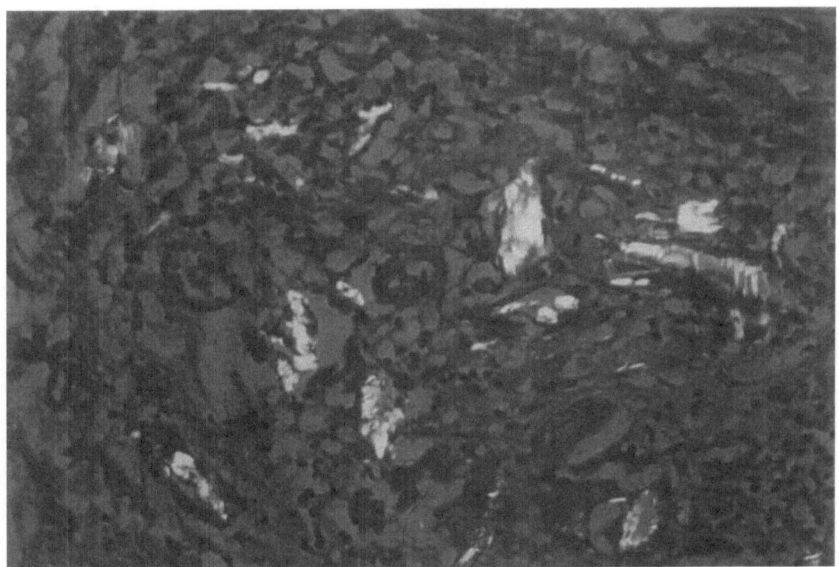

Figure 179 The same field as in Figure 178 reveals the presence of doubly-refractile material within clefts that are situated in the tumour (× 275)

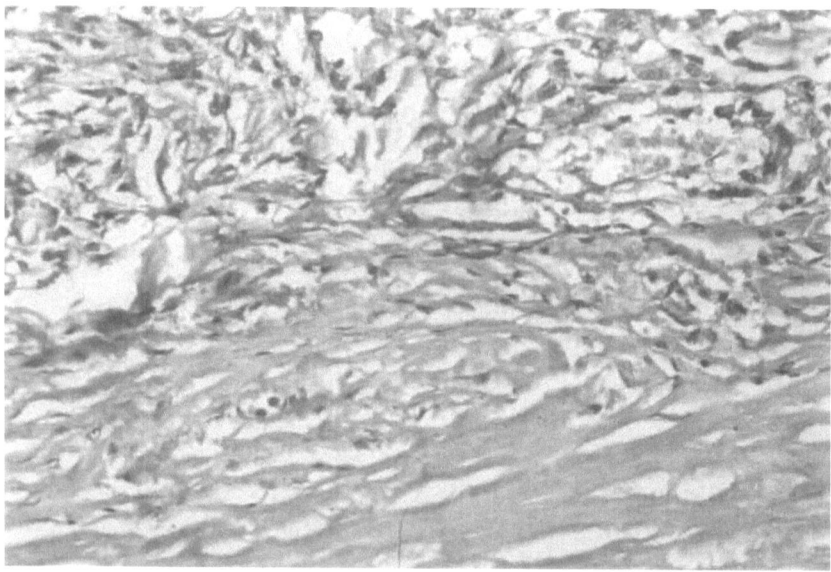

Figure 180   The border zone between the tumour and the plaque shows similar clefts and reaction, as seen in Figures 178 and 179 (× 275)

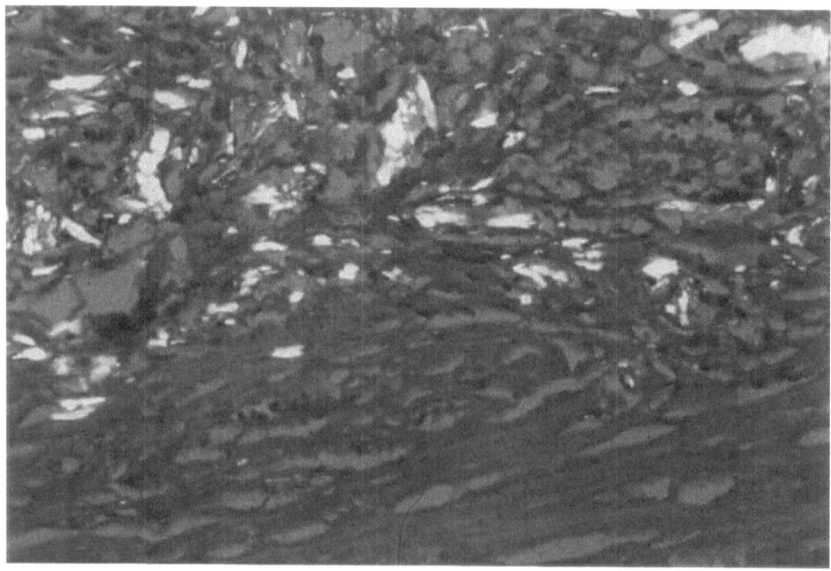

Figure 181   The same field as in Figure 180 showing doubly-refractile material (× 275)

Case No. 5
Diffuse malignant mesothelioma of the pericardium

Clinical history

A 53-year-old man. For ten years he had symptoms of angina pectoris, accompanied for the last two years by functional dyspnoea. An E.C.G. tracing in 1968 revealed a low voltage pattern. No signs of heart failure were present.

He was re-admitted to hospital in 1970 with signs of severe heart failure and atrial fibrillation. E.C.G. showed a more pronounced low voltage pattern and iso-electric T waves. Chest x-ray showed cardiac enlargement but the contour was normal. He died rapidly with increasing cardiac failure.

Occupational history

The patient had worked in the tobacco industry. There was no history of asbestos exposure.

Autopsy findings

The pericardial cavity was distended and contained 70 ml of blood-stained fluid. The parietal pericardium was thickened (between 3 mm and 8 mm) and the visceral pericardium was also thickened (between 6 mm and 27 mm). Both layers were infiltrated by a grey-white tumour with the consistency of cartilage. The tumour totally encased the heart. The surface of the tumour was nodular and there was only shallow infiltration into the underlying myocardium. The coronary arteries contained only small amounts of atheroma. There were metastatic tumour deposits in the mediastinal lymph nodes, including those in the carinal and peri-tracheal region. No other tumour deposits were present in any organ, and in particular there was no tumour involving the pleura or peritoneum. Bilateral pleural effusions were present and there was a small pulmonary infarct. Chronic congestive changes were present in the lungs. Microscopy showed features of a typical mesothelioma.

Acknowledgement

This case was kindly contributed by Dr Johan Adolf Andersen (Andersen, J.A. and Hansen, B.F. (1974). Mesothelioma of the pericardium. *Ugeskr. Læger*, **136,** 150–3)

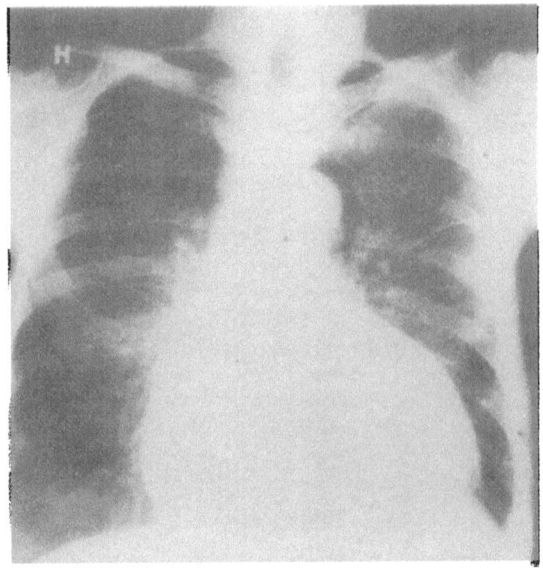

Figure 182 P.A. view of chest shows an enlarged, but otherwise normal heart

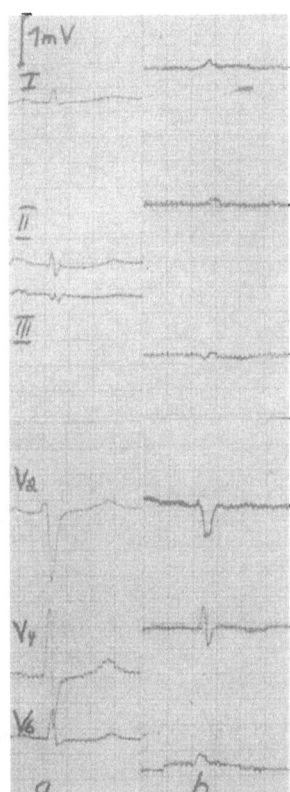

Figure 183 E.C.G.
tracing (a) taken in
November 1968 and (b)
taken in November
1970. Note the more
pronounced low voltage
pattern and the
appearance of iso-
electric T waves in the
latter tracing

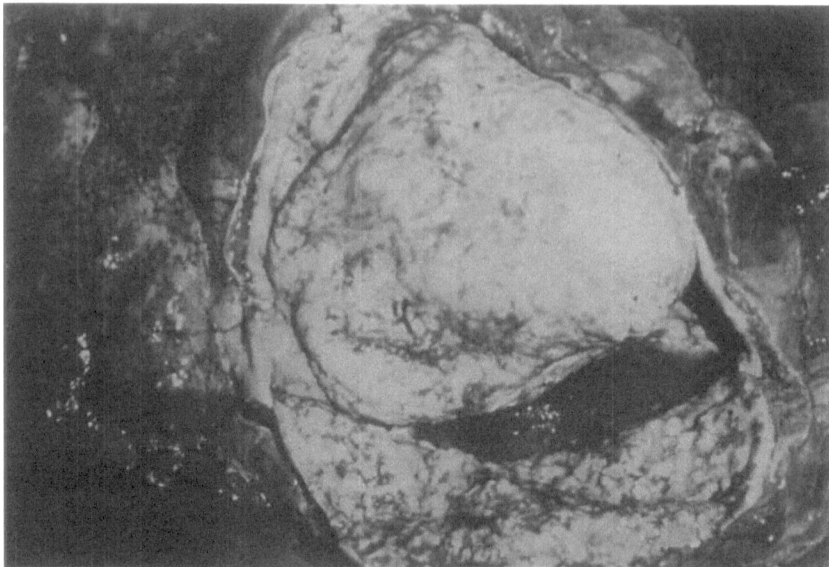

Figure 184 Autopsy specimen of the pericardium opened *in situ*. Both the parietal and visceral layers of the pericardium are diffusely infiltrated by white nodular tissue. The thickness varies from 5 to 25 mm. On both sides of the heart the pleura is seen to be normal

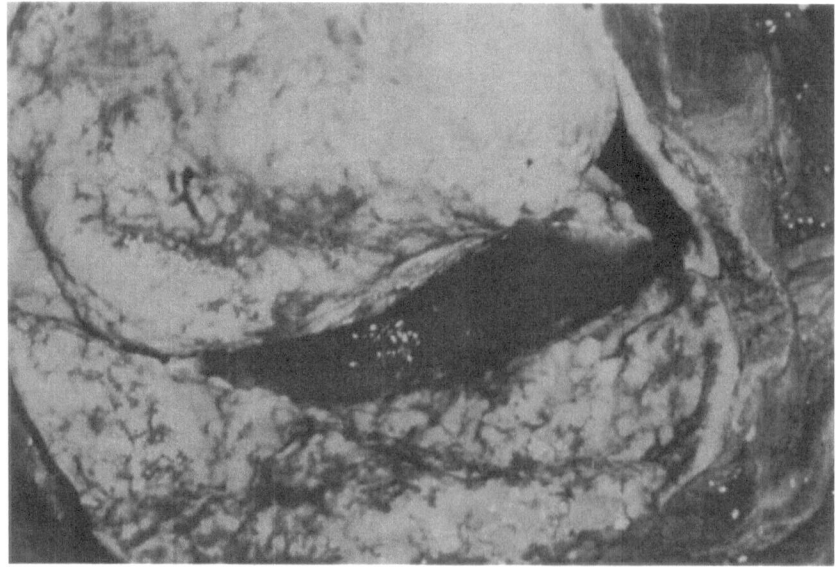

Figure 185 A localized area of pericardium to show the details of Figure 184

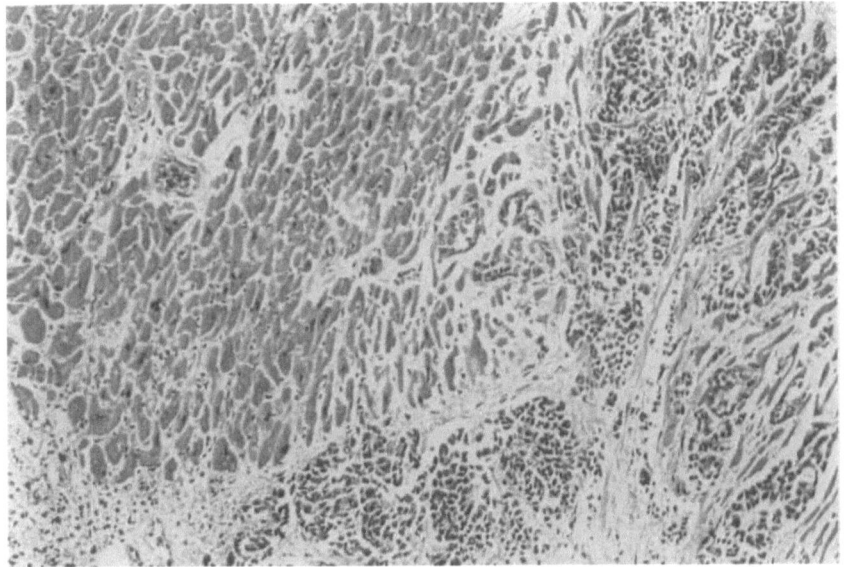

Figure 186 The tumour is seen to spread over the surface of the pericardium (× 110)

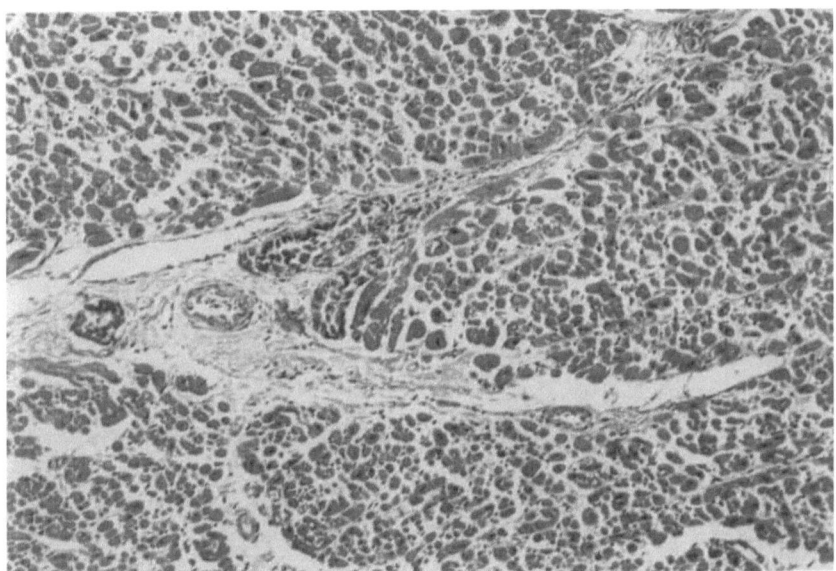

Figure 187 Tumour has spread into perivascular tissue within the myocardium (× 110)

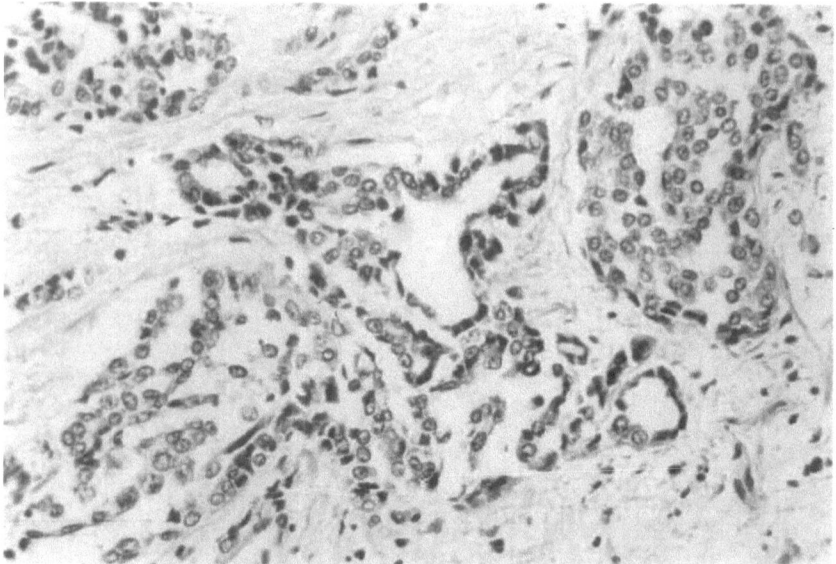

Figure 188   The pericardial tumour shows a tubular pattern with a lining of non-mucin-secreting cuboidal cells situated in a loose connective tissue stroma (× 275)

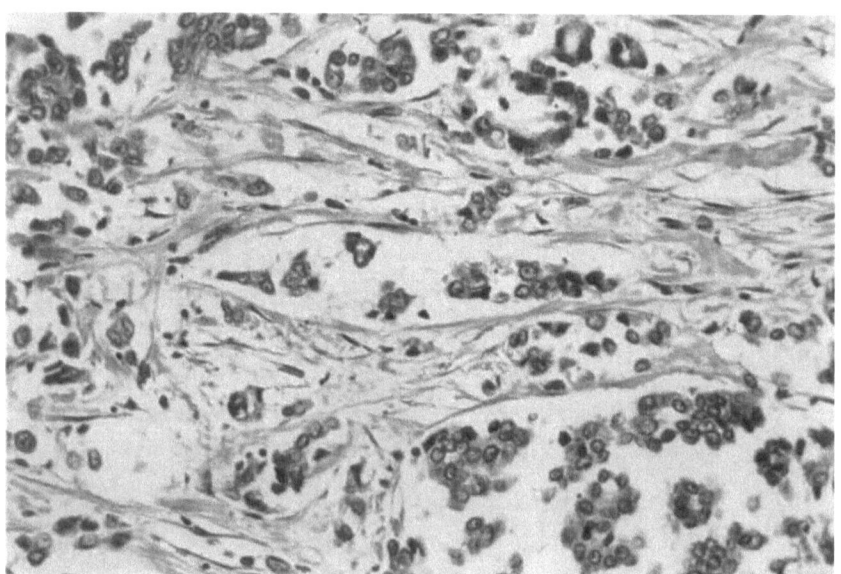

Figure 189   This area shows a mixture of epithelial and connective tissue elements (× 275)

Case No. 6
Diffuse malignant mesothelioma of the pleura – mixed type

Clinical history

A 75-year-old man. He developed Horner's syndrome on the right side in September 1981. He also showed signs of involvement of the brachial plexus accompanied by pain in his right arm. X-ray of the thorax showed a shadow at the apex of the right lung. Though malignancy was not confirmed by biopsy the lesion was irradiated in October. The pain grew worse and the patient's condition deteriorated. He died in November 1981.

Occupational history

Had worked in a shipyard.

Autopsy findings

A tumour of 7 cm diameter was found low in the right neck. It was fixed to the apex of the lung and to the vertebral column. The visceral and parietal pleurae on the right side showed several flat tumours of maximum diameter 3 cm. Multiple pleural plaques were found on both sides. No metastases were present.

Microscopy showed the tumour to be a mesothelioma mainly of connnective tissue type. An epithelial component was found in some places only. Many asbestos bodies were present in the lung tissue.

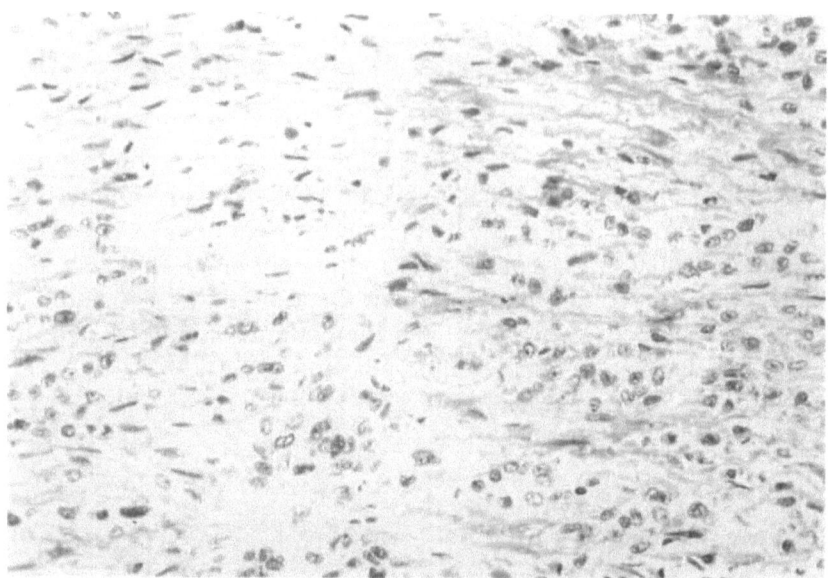

Figure 190   A connective tissue type of tumour with areas showing moderate amounts of fibrillar collagen ($\times$ 275)

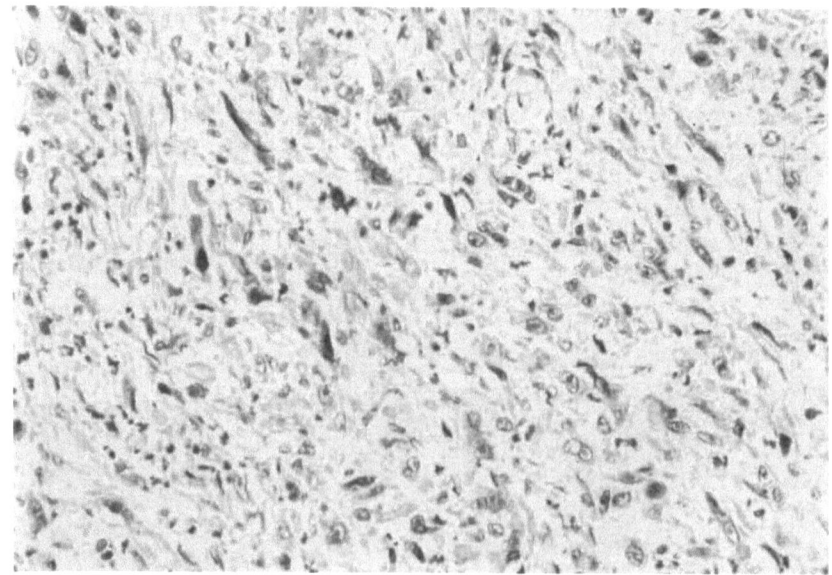

Figure 191   A more pleomorphic field ($\times$ 275)

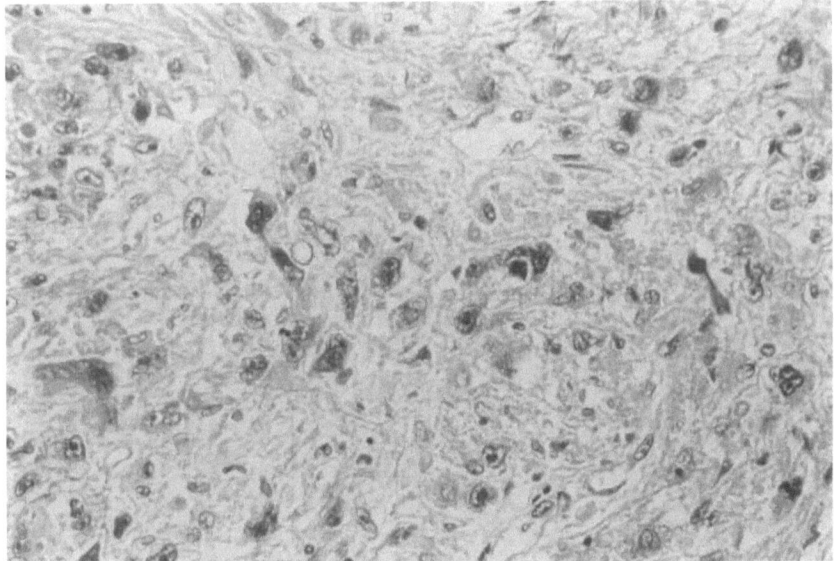

Figure 192 A highly pleomorphic area, but still of connective tissue type (× 275)

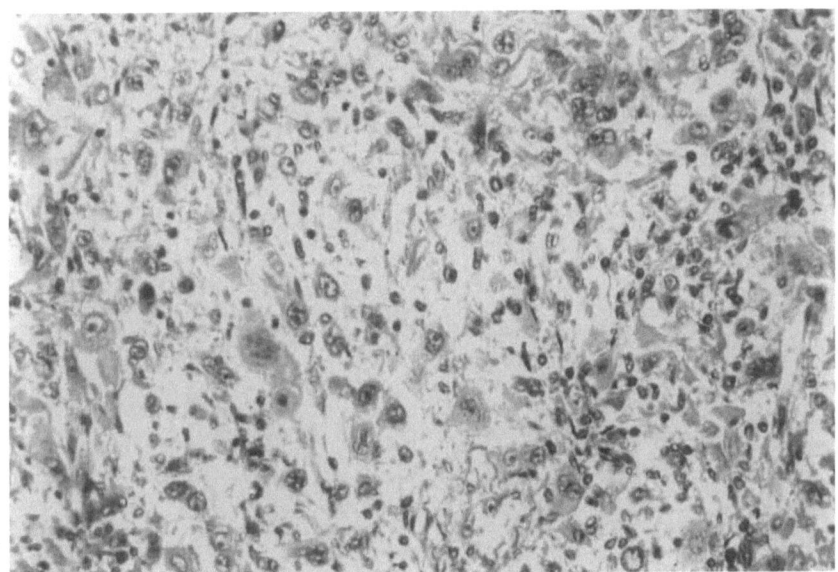

Figure 193 A looser arrangement of tumour cells which are more rounded and epithelial like. There is a moderate lymphocytic infiltration (× 275)

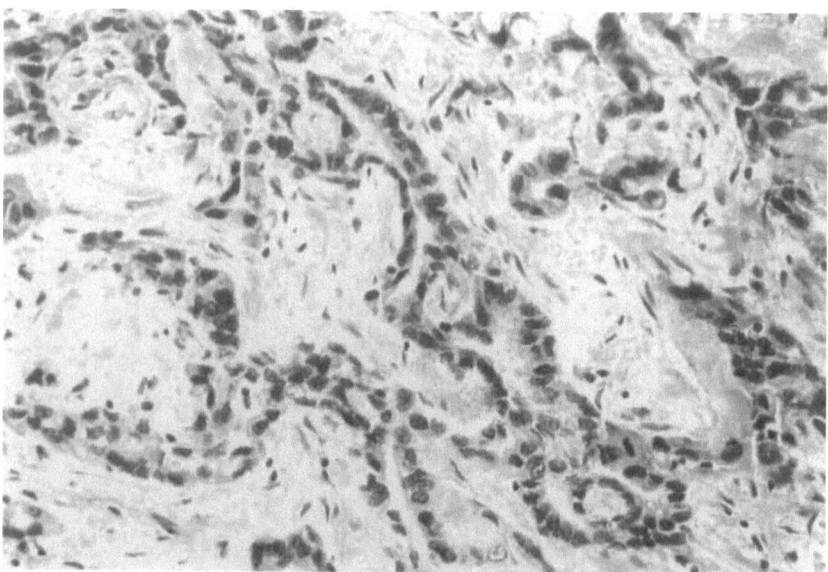

Figure 194 A completely different pattern from the previous figures, dominated by tubules lined by a single layer of epithelial type cells (× 275)

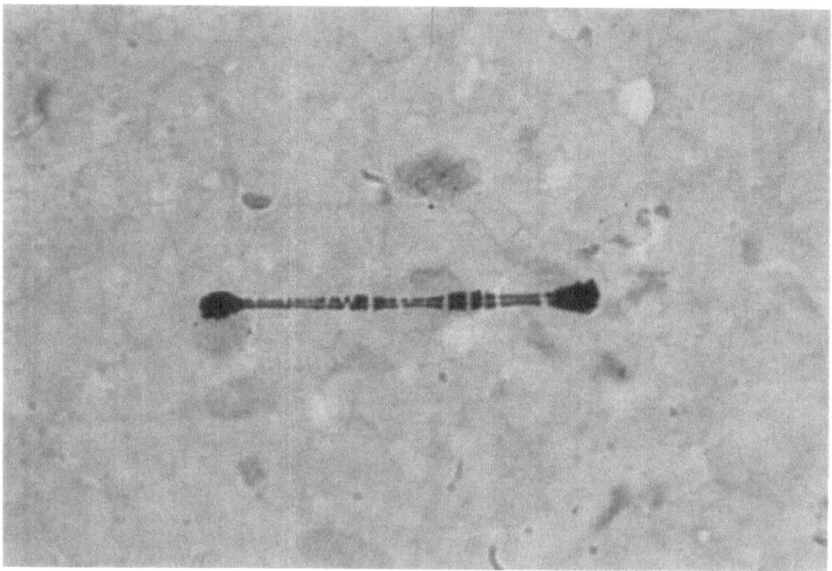

Figure 195 An imprint preparation from the cut surface of the lung, revealing an asbestos body. Perl's iron stain (× 730)

Case No. 7
Asbestosis and carcinoma (with mesothelioma?)

Clinical history

A 43-year-old man. He was admitted to hospital in 1975 when a diagnosis of asbestosis was made. Two years later he was suspected of having a malignant tumour in the left lung. In December 1979 a left sided pneumonectomy was carried out but it was known that some pleural tumour was not completely removed.

The patient died in October 1980.

Occupational history

The patient worked as an insulator in a shipyard for more than 15 years, during which time he had heavy asbestos exposure.

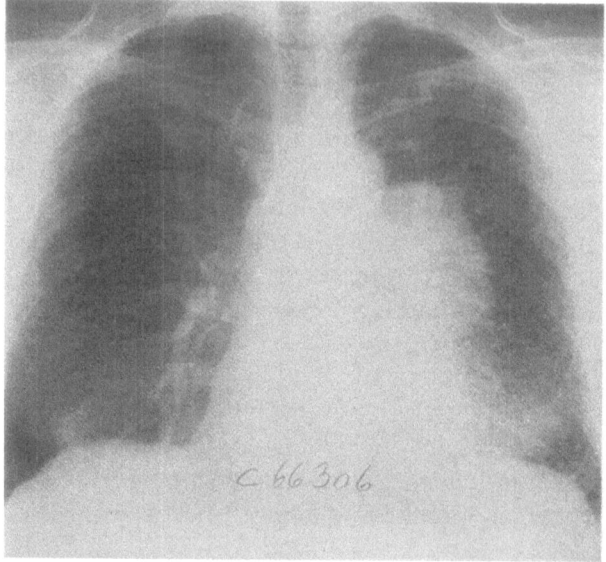

Figure 196   A preoperative P.A. view of chest shows a
dense opacity at left hilum and diffuse shadowing of both
lower lobes. There is doubtful thickening of the left pleura

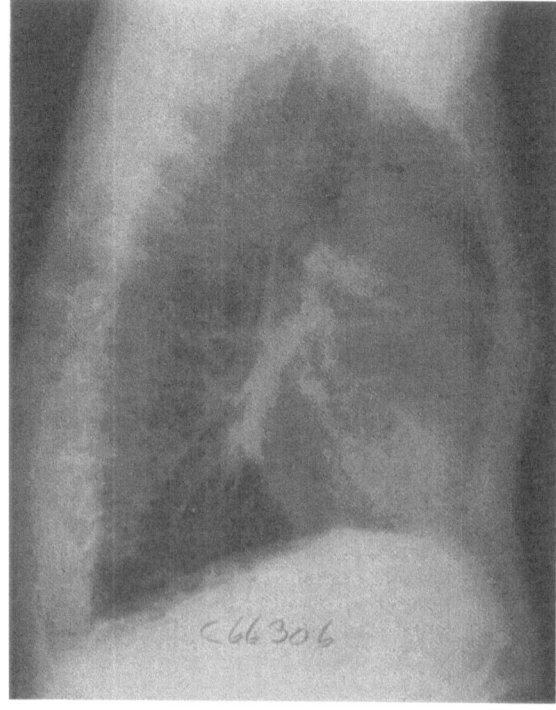

Figure 197   A lateral view of above

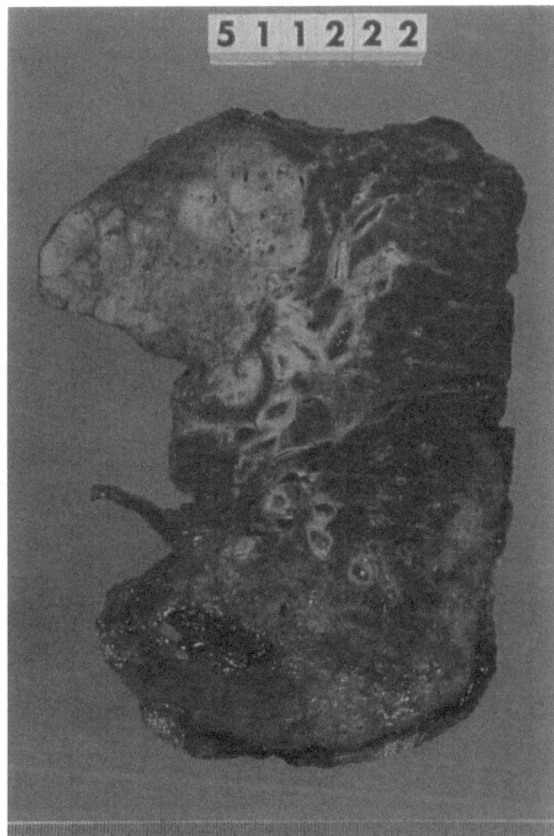

Figure 198 Left pneumonectomy specimen shows a large tumour mass above the hilum and a more diffuse tumour infiltration of the lower lobe. Tumour is also present in the pleura at the lower part of the specimen. The lung parenchyma is shrunken at the costo-phrenic angle

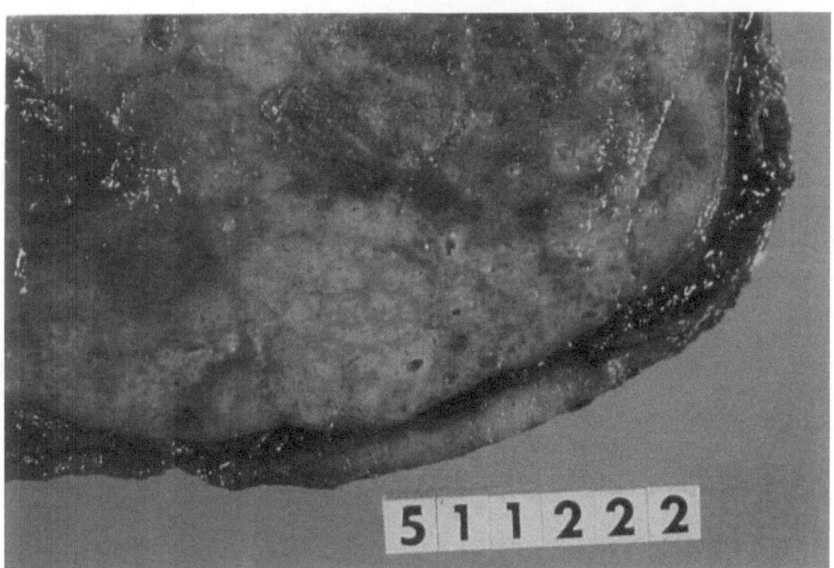

Figure 199 A more detailed view to show the tumour infiltration of the pleura, separated from the pulmonary tumour

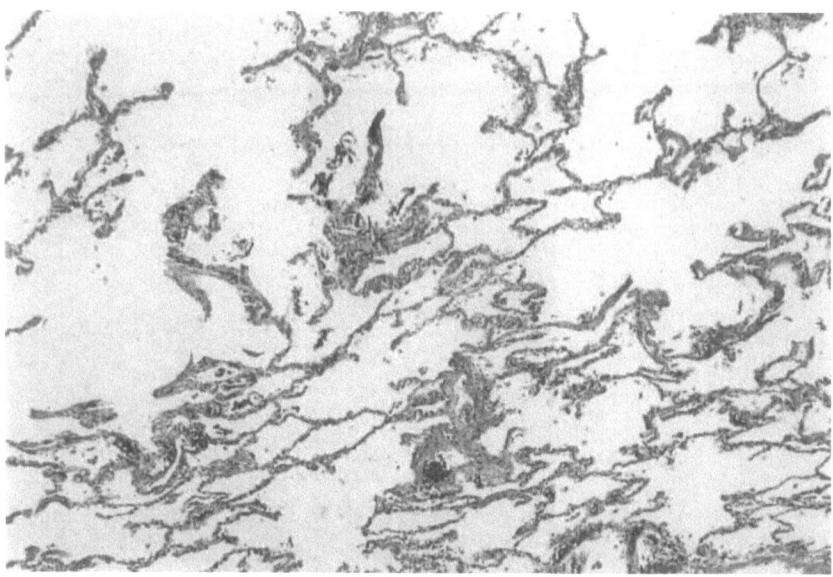

Figure 200 Low magnification to show asbestosis (× 45)

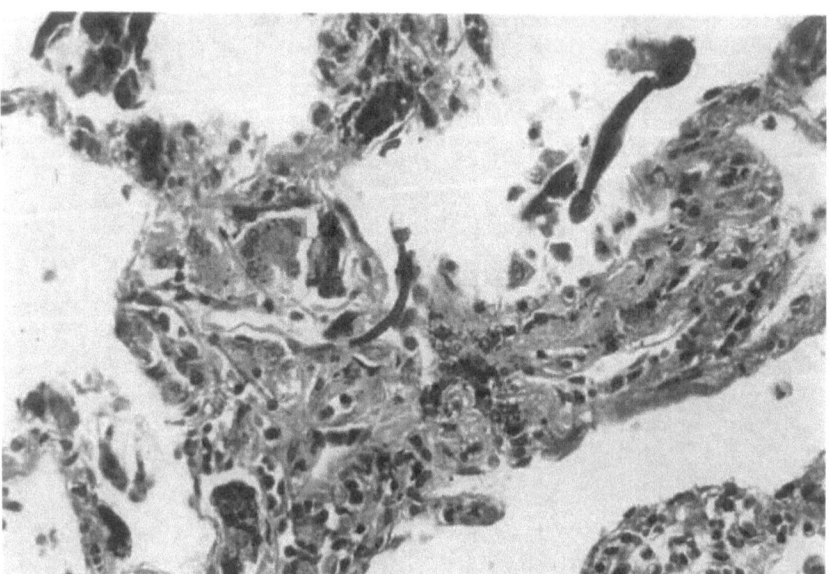

Figure 201 Higher magnification of the same field to show fibrosis and asbestos bodies (× 275)

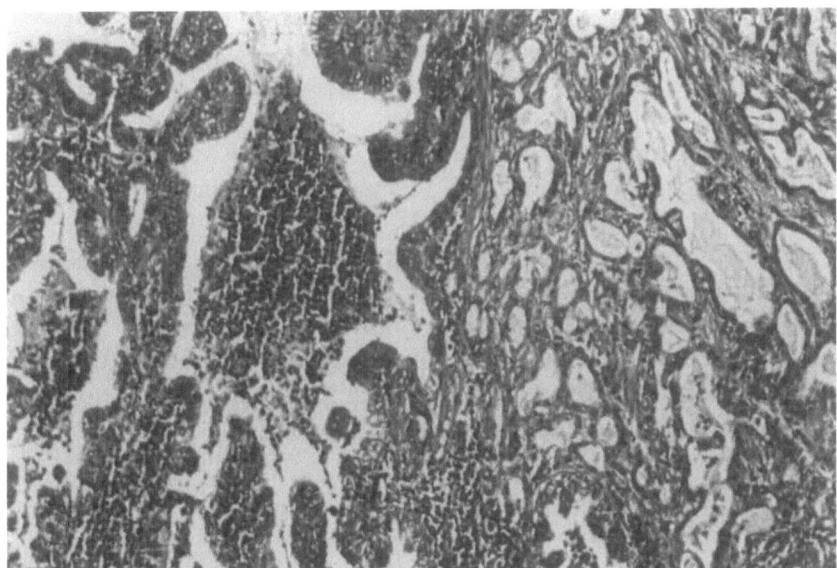

Figure 202 On the left half of the figure there is a well differentiated adenocarcinoma. On the right half there is a tubular, microcystic tumour with a lining of flattened cells (× 110)

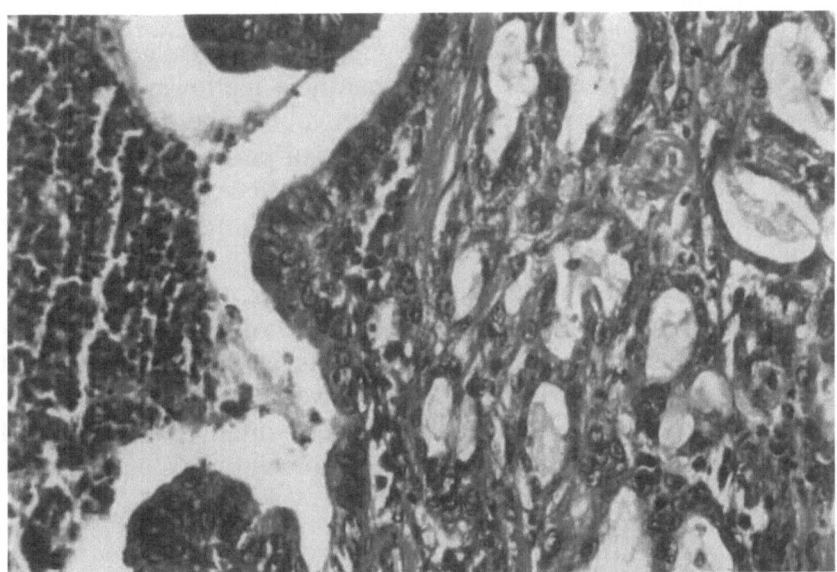

Figure 203 A higher power view of the same field shows the two different tumour types. The question posed is whether there are two types of adenocarcinoma present, or whether the tumour on the left is an adenocarcinoma, and the tumour on the right is a mesothelioma of epithelial type? The diastase–PAS and alcian blue stains were strongly positive for the tumour on the left. In the tumour cells on the right, they were negative, but the material in the tubules was weakly positive. While it is probable that both tumour types are variants of an adenocarcinoma, the possibility of a co-existing mesothelioma cannot be excluded (compare with a different patient illustrated in Figures 78–81) (× 275)

Case No. 8
Cystic mesothelioma of the peritoneum

Clinical history

A 36-year-old man. He was admitted to hospital with a swelling in the right iliac fossa. Laparotomy revealed a large mass of cysts in the region of the appendix. The mass was removed. Four years later he was readmitted and it was found that his abdominal cavity was filled with multiple cysts. These arose on the surface of all organs and on the peritoneal surface of the abdominal wall. Biopsies revealed cystic mesothelioma, histologically identical to the earlier lesion. The patient is alive and well at the latest follow up examination nine months after the second laparotomy.

Occupational history

The patient was a shipyard worker from the age of 16 to 29 years. He worked with asbestos materials throughout his employment.

Characteristics

Cystic mesothelioma consists of multiple thin-walled cysts of variable sizes. It is situated predominantly in the lower part of the peritoneal cavity and it is commonest in young adult females. This lesion has not been reported in the pleura or pericardium. The biological behaviour of the small number of reported cases is in keeping with the lesion being a mesothelioma of either borderline type or of very low grade malignancy.

Histologically there are collections of cysts, tubules and clefts, lined by a single layer of mesothelial-like cells which may range from columnar to flattened. Those microcysts which are lined by flattened cells may be confused with fat cells. However the content of the cysts is alcian-blue positive. The cuboidal cells often have a hobnail appearance. The connective tissue component may be loose or dense.

Acknowledgement

This case was kindly contributed by Professor I. Taylor and Dr G.H. Millward-Sadler.

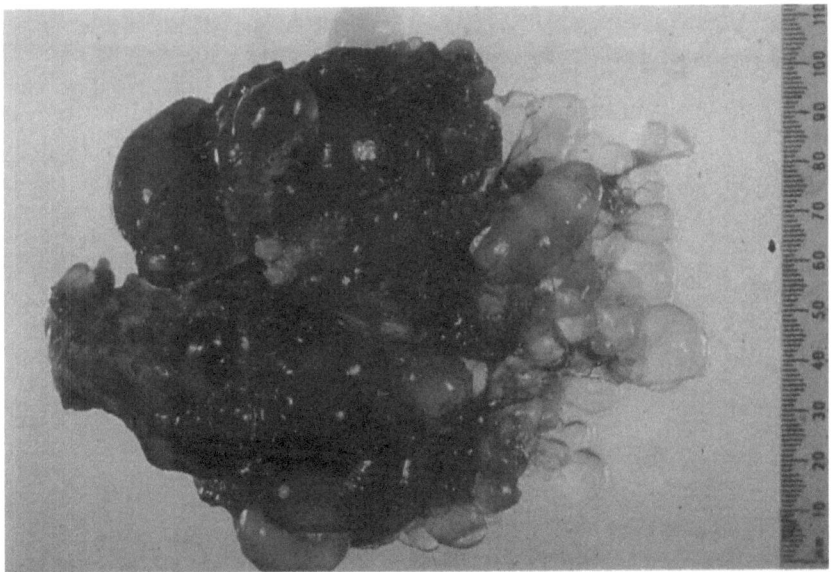

Figure 204 Cystic mass removed at laparotomy

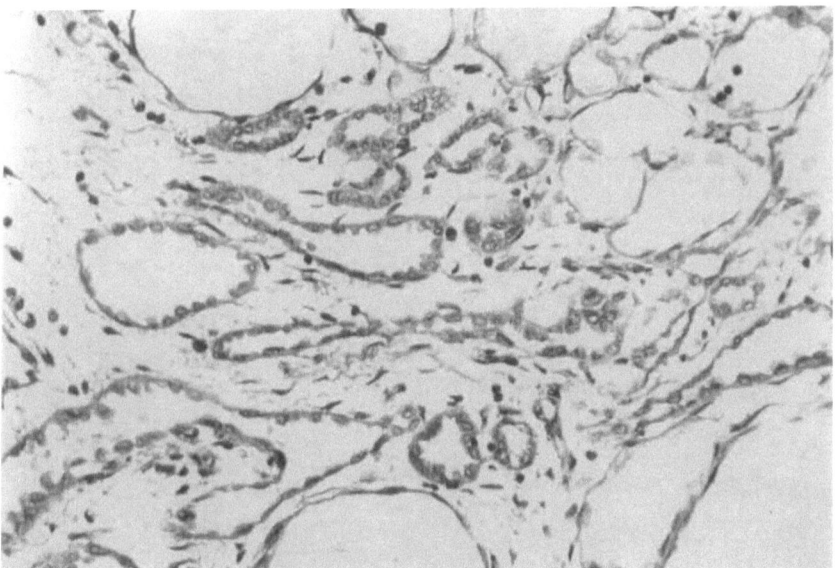

Figure 205 Microscopic appearance of above showing clefts, tubules and microcysts irregularly arranged in a loose connective tissue. Even at this magnification prominence of the nuclei is apparent – the so called hobnail appearance. (× 275)

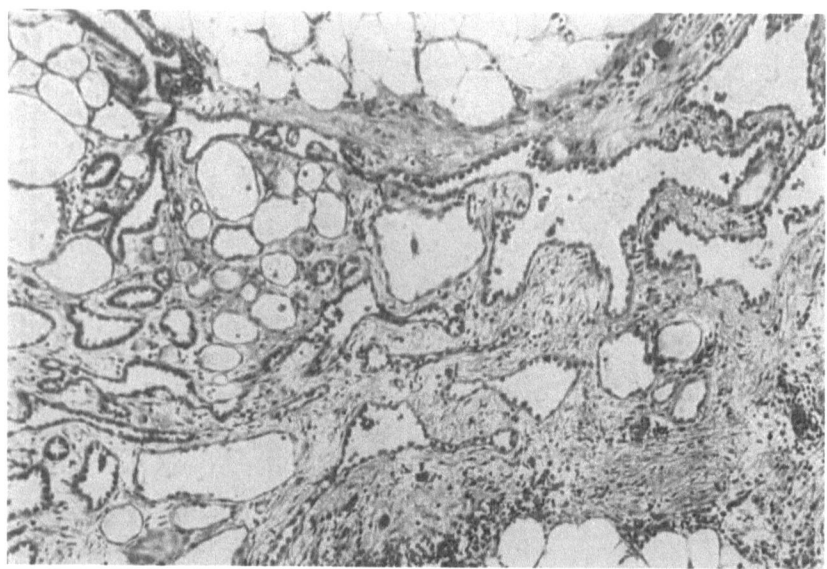

Figure 206   Clefts, tubules and microcysts with dense connective tissue seen in the centre (× 110)

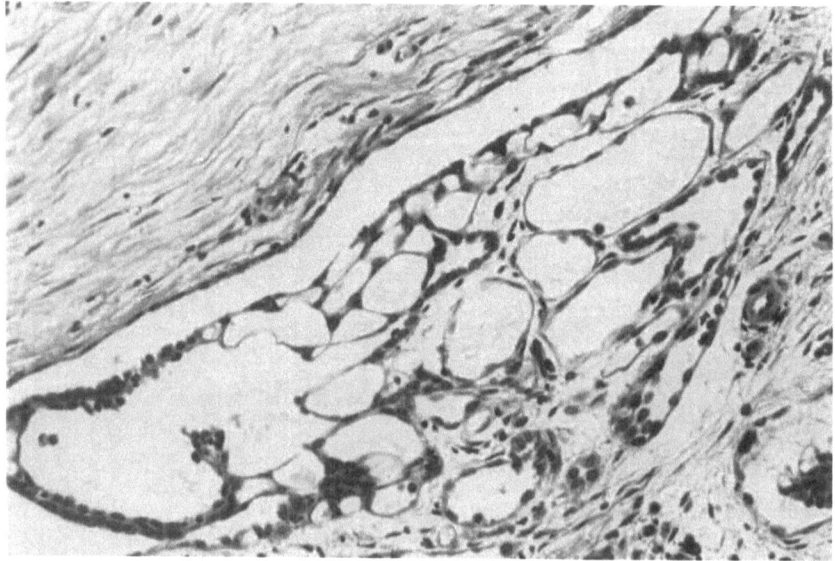

Figure 207   Higher power view of a similar area (× 275)

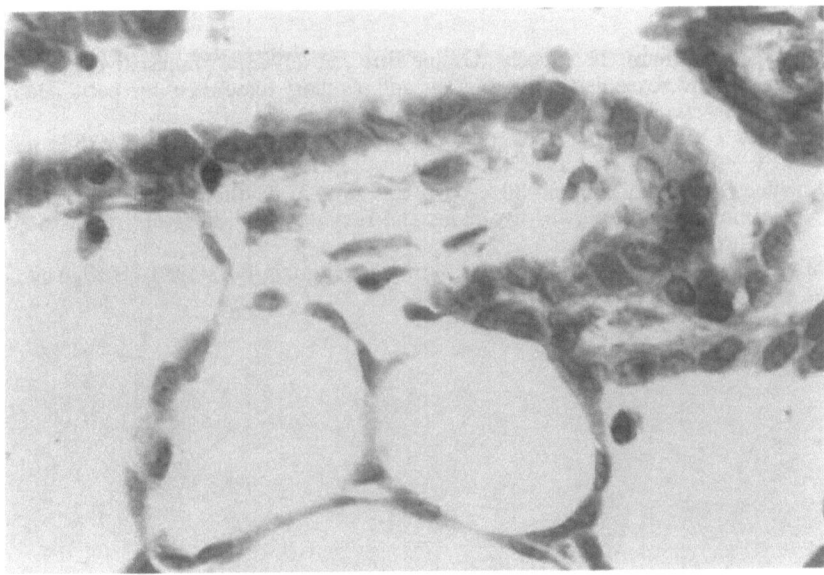

Figure 208 High power view showing the regular lining of columnar cells of a tubule (top) and flattened cells lining microcysts (bottom) (× 730)

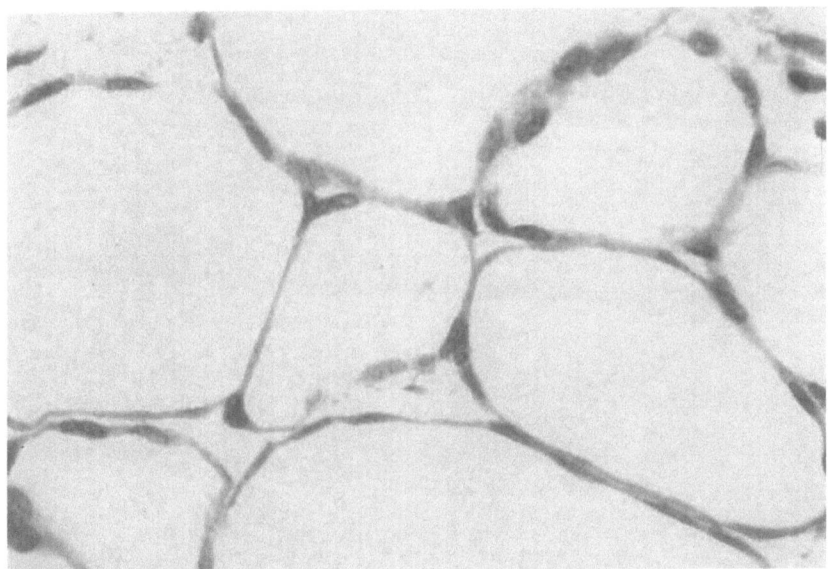

Figure 209 Microcysts lined by flattened cells, mimicking fat cells (× 730)

References

Dumke, K., Schnoy, N., Specht, G. and Buse, H. (1983). Comparative light and electron microscopic studies of cystic and papillary tumours of the peritoneum. *Virch.Arch. (Pathol. Anat.)*, **399**, 25–39

Enzinger, F.M. and Weiss, S.W. (1983). *Soft Tissue Tumors*. pp. 571–574 (St Louis: C.V. Mosby)

Katsube, Y., Mukai, K. and Silverberg, S.G. (1982). Cystic mesothelioma of the peritoneum. A report of five cases and review of the literature. *Cancer,* **50**, 1615–1622

Moore, J.H., Crum, C.P., Chandler, J.E. and Feldman, P.S. (1980). Benign cystic mesothelioma. *Cancer*, **45**, 2395–2399

4

Other forms of Mesothelioma

I. BENIGN LOCALIZED MESOTHELIOMA OF PLEURA

Synonyms:
Localized fibrous mesothelioma.
Solitary fibrous tumour of the pleura.
Benign local pleural fibroma.
Submesothelial fibroma.
Localised solitary monophasic spindle-cell tumour.
Leiomyofibroma.
Endothelioma.

Age range:
From 3rd to 7th decade, with a peak incidence in the 5th and 6th decade.

Symptoms and signs:
The clinical presentation ranges from silent opacities on chest x-ray to severe dyspnoea. Localized pain and a feeling of a foreign body in the chest may occur. Extrapulmonary symptoms such as osteo-arthritis and rheumatoid arthritis may be encountered, as well as hypoglycaemia. Exposure to asbestos or other mineral fibres are not features. The patient is nearly always fully cured after radical surgery.
A few deaths have been recorded due to extensive intrathoracic growth, either caused by late diagnosis or by an unresectable recurrence.

Gross pathology: The tumour is characteristically located in the pleural cavity and attached to the visceral pleura by a thin stalk. The surface is smooth and although the tumour may nearly fill the whole pleural cavity there is no infiltration into neighbouring tissues. The cut surface is firm and shows a whorled pattern. Calcification ·and cysts occur, but necrosis and haemorrhage are rare.

Histopathology: The tumour is composed of spindle cells in a whorled arrangement, often forming interlacing bundles alternating with a cellular-poor area, dominated by reticulin and collagen fibres with a varying degree of hyalinization. Small clefts lined by mesothelial-like cells may predominate. The microscopic picture varies from area to area and from tumour to tumour. A few cases with a sarcomatous morphology, cellular pleomorphism and a high number of mitoses, have been described. Even in these cases there seems to be a good prognosis if a pedicle is present.

Histogenesis: It is still under debate whether the tumour should be considered a true mesothelioma or whether it is derived from submesothelial connective tissue.

Case history: A 77-year-old man. He developed increasing dyspnoea. A large tumour ($12 \times 8 \times 6$ cm) compressed the right lung. It was found to be attached to the lower lobe region by a thin stalk and it was surgically removed. The patient made an uneventful recovery.

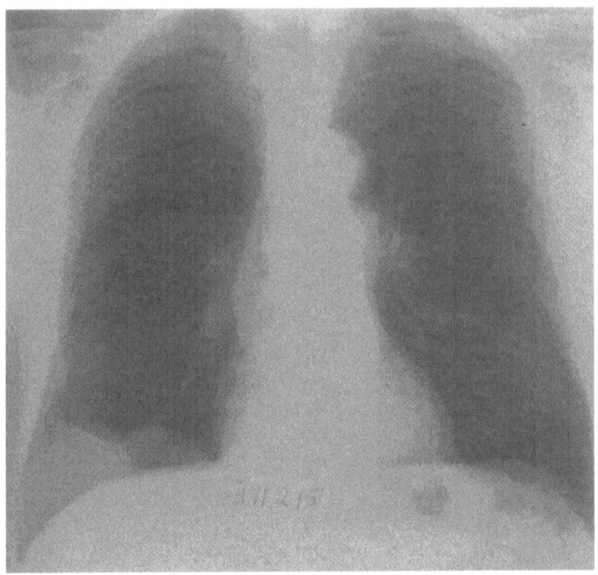

Figure 210   P.A. view of chest to show sharply demarcated opacity in the right costo-phrenic angle

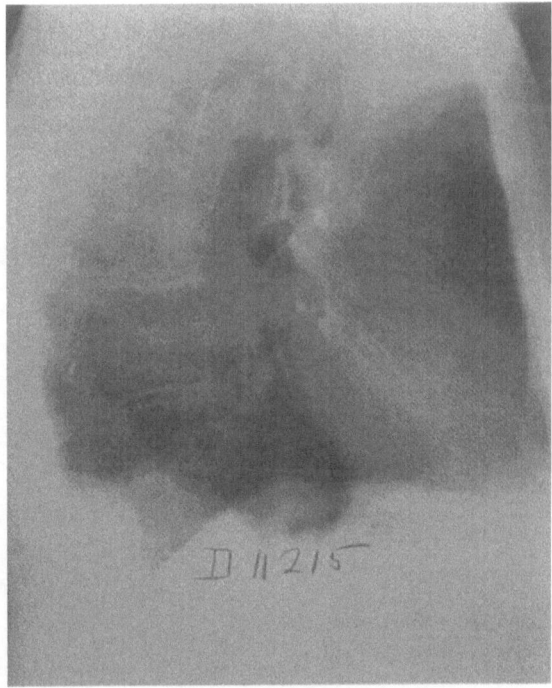

Figure 211   Oblique view of the above indicating the posterior position of the opacity

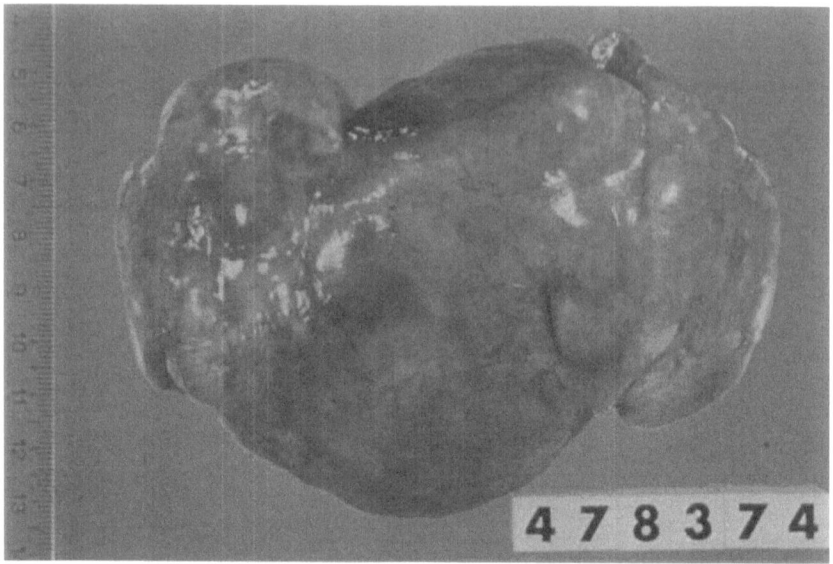

Figure 212   Surgically resected specimen of the solitary pedunculated pleural tumour. There is a smooth nodular surface, and the capsule is intact

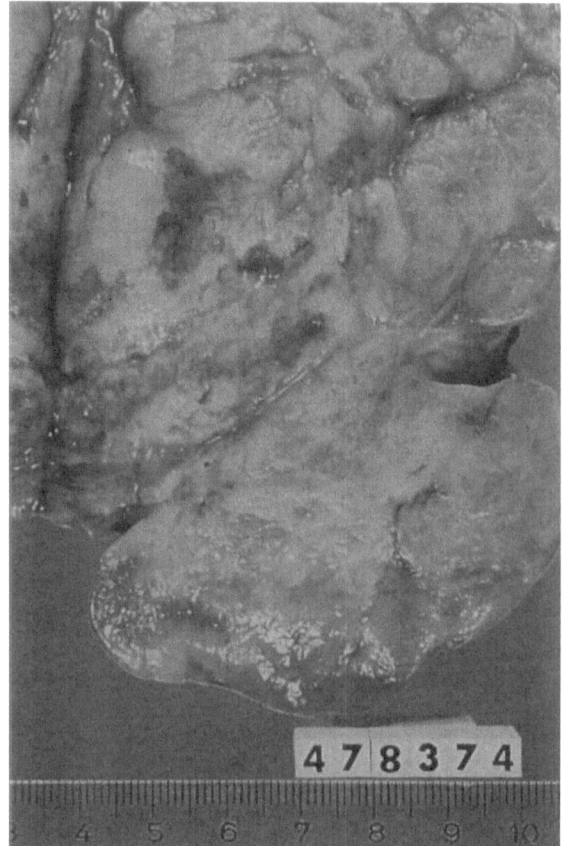

Figure 213   The cut surface shows a whorled pattern

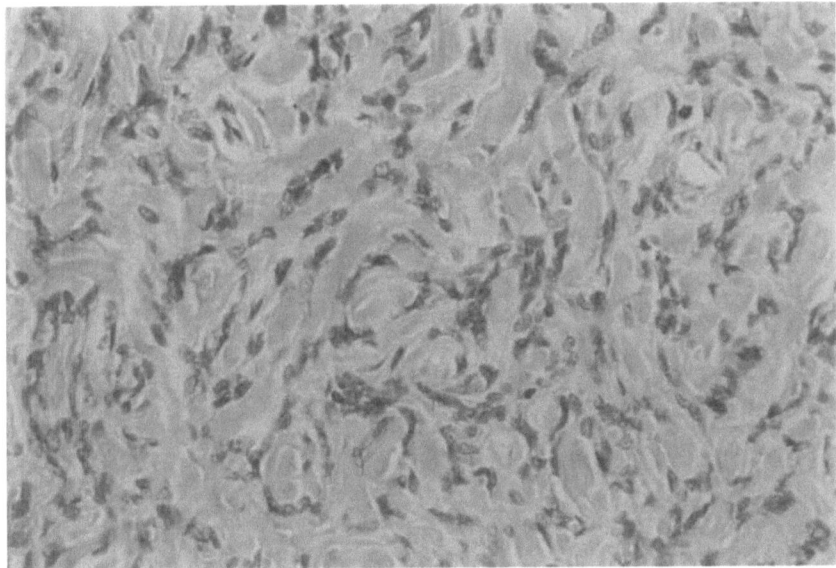

Figure 214 The characteristic feature of this tumour is seen here as coarse bundles of interwoven collagen. The nuclei are rather blunt and are often seen to be in the clefts between the collagen (× 275)

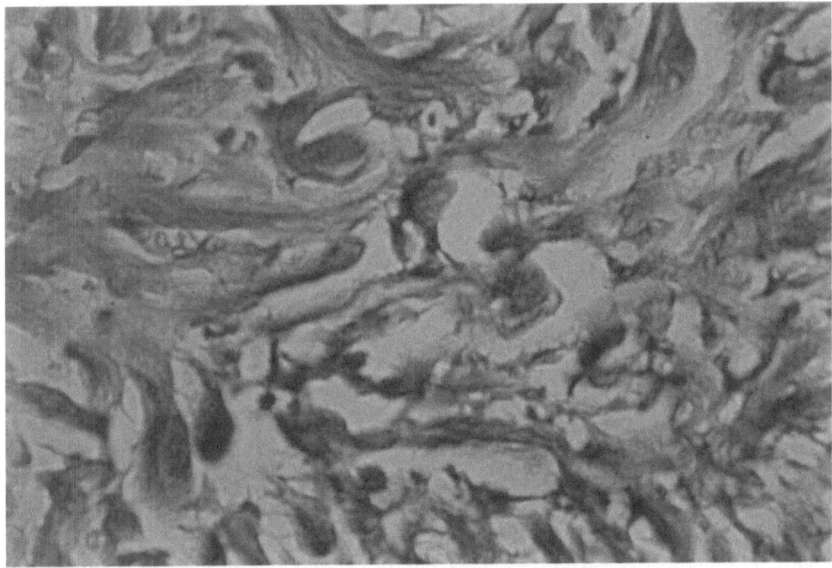

Figure 215 Van Gieson-stained section of the above (× 430)

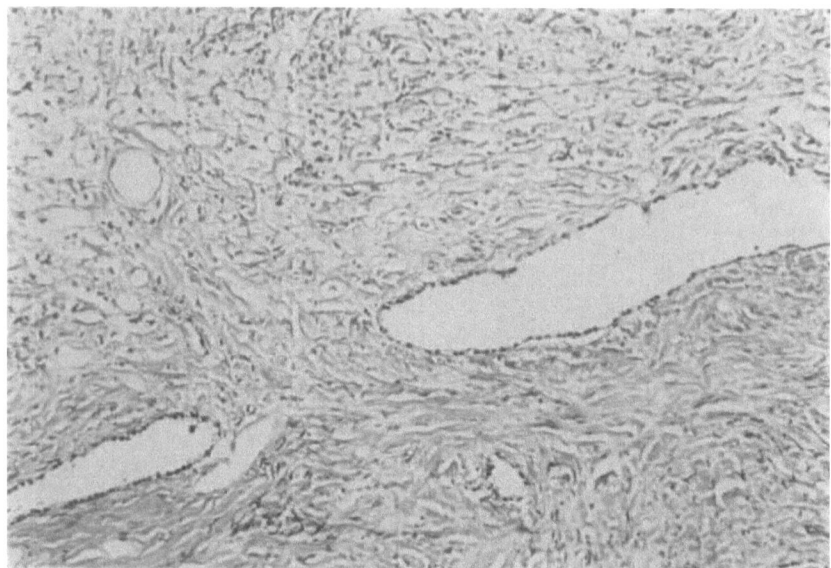

Figure 216   Less characteristic features of this tumour are seen as clefts lined by a single layer of flattened mesothelial-like cells (× 110)

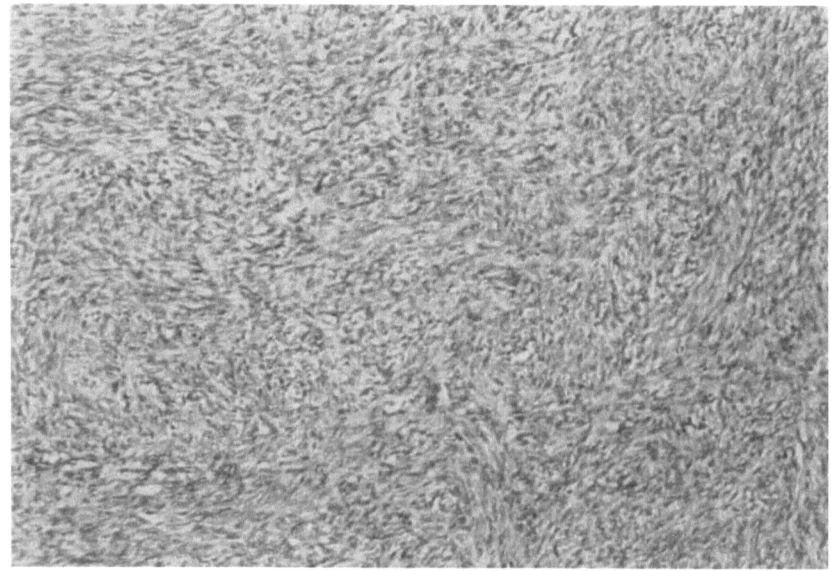

Figure 217   Another variant shows a highly cellular appearance with interlacing bundles of spindle cells (× 110)

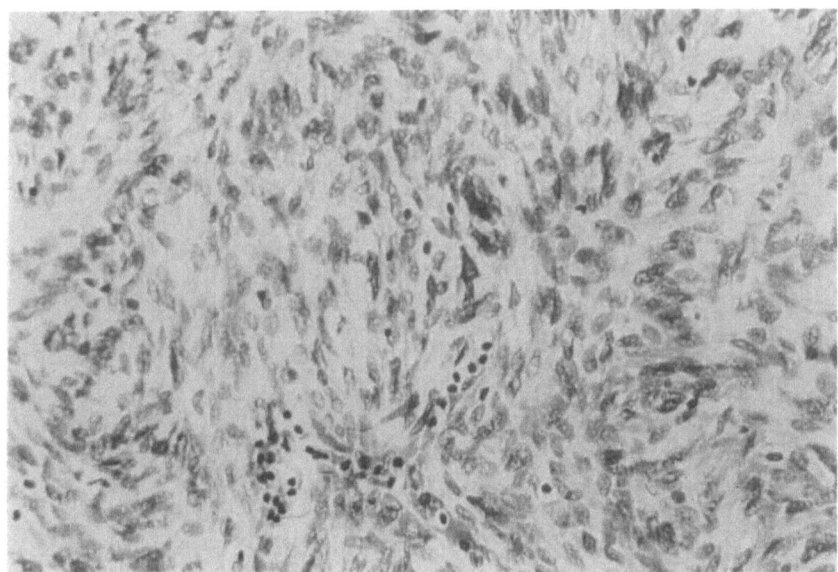

Figure 218 A further variant shows a more pleomorphic picture with scattered lymphocytes (× 275)

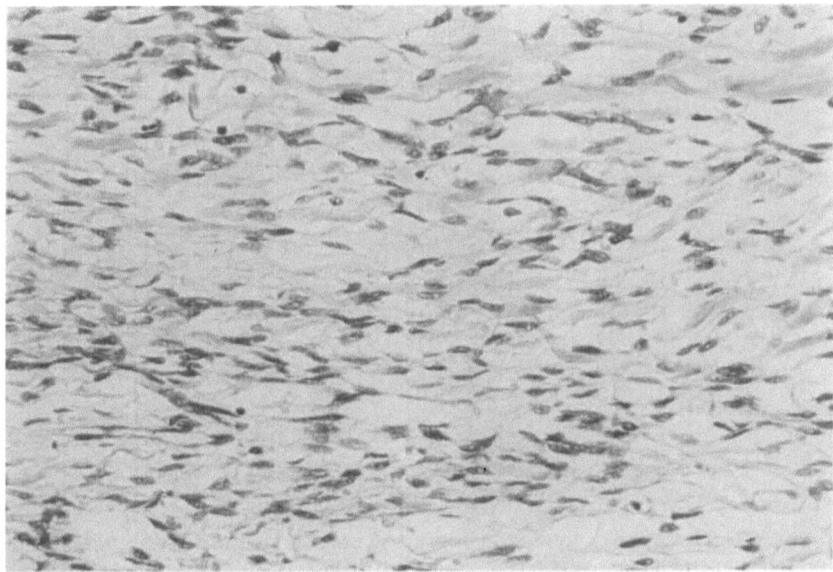

Figure 219 A more wavy arrangement of cells may be seen (× 275)

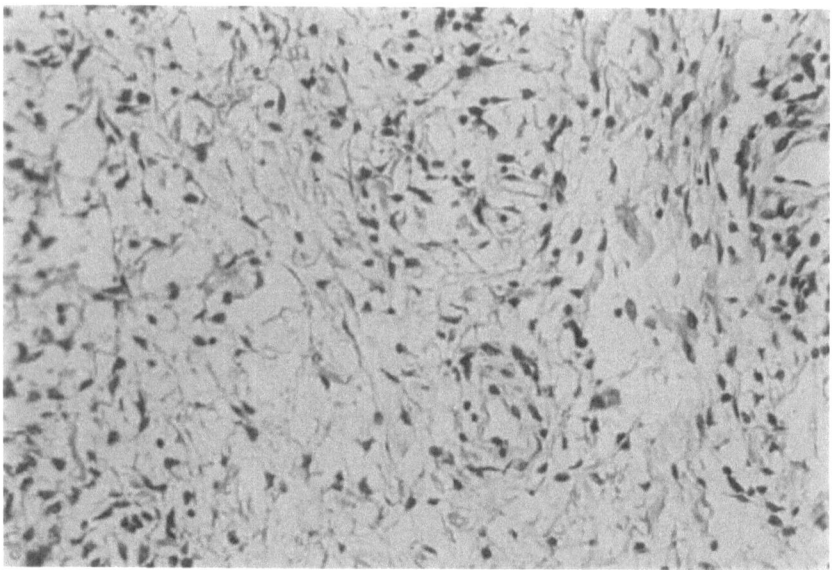

Figure 220   A loose structure with a myxoid appearance features in this tumour (× 275)

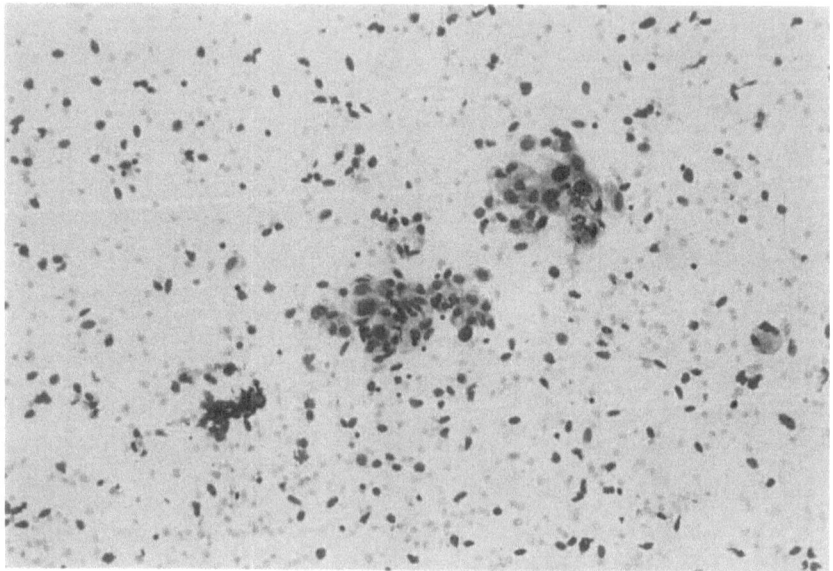

Figure 221   Low power view of an imprint. A constant feature of this tumour is the presence of small cigar-shaped separate cells. Clusters of large epithelial-like cells may also be seen. May-Grünwald-Giemsa stain (× 110)

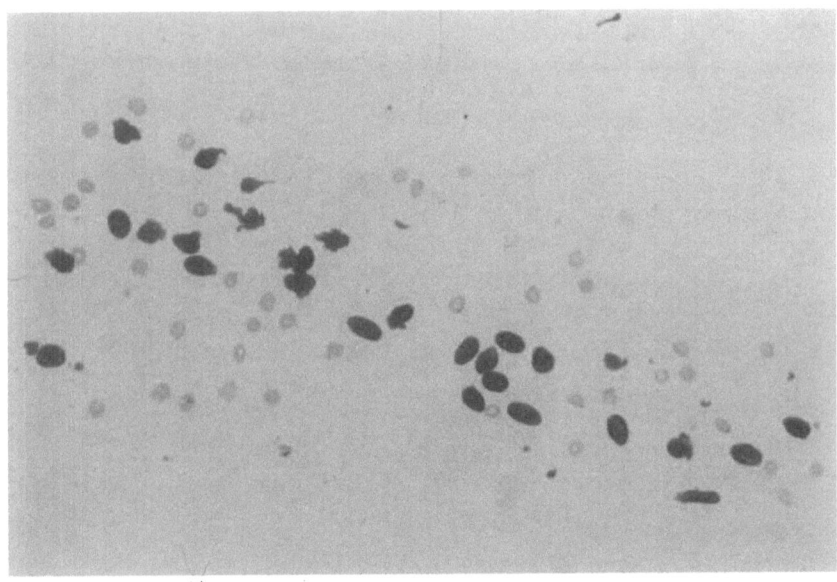

Figure 222   A higher power view of the small cigar-shaped nuclei, which are typical of benign connective tissue type cells. May-Grünwald-Giemsa stain (× 275)

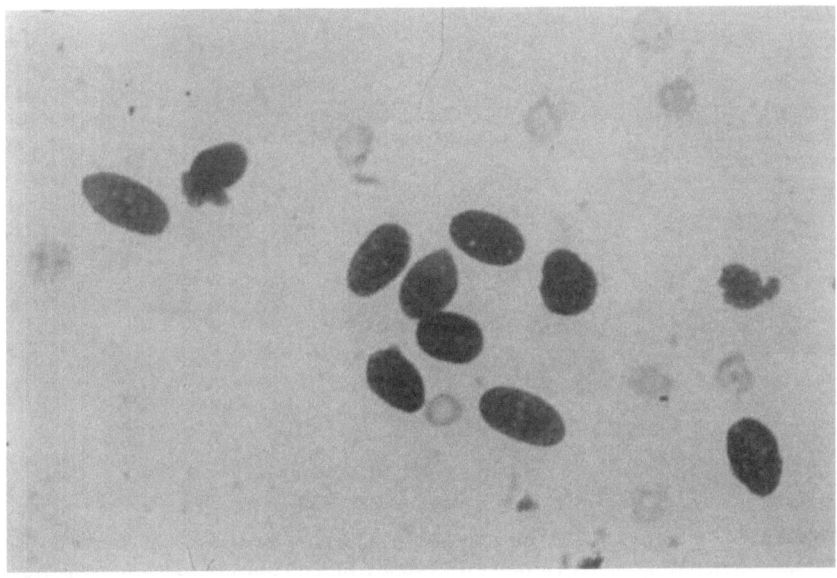

Figure 223   A high power view of the same cells. May-Grünwald-Giemsa stain (× 800)

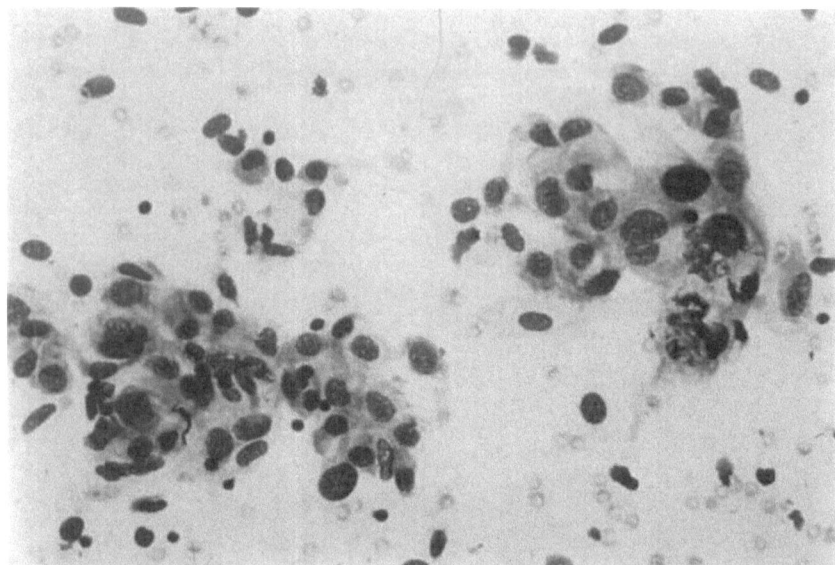

Figure 224 The larger epithelial-like cells show rather abundant, pale cytoplasm. May-Grünwald-Giemsa stain (× 275)

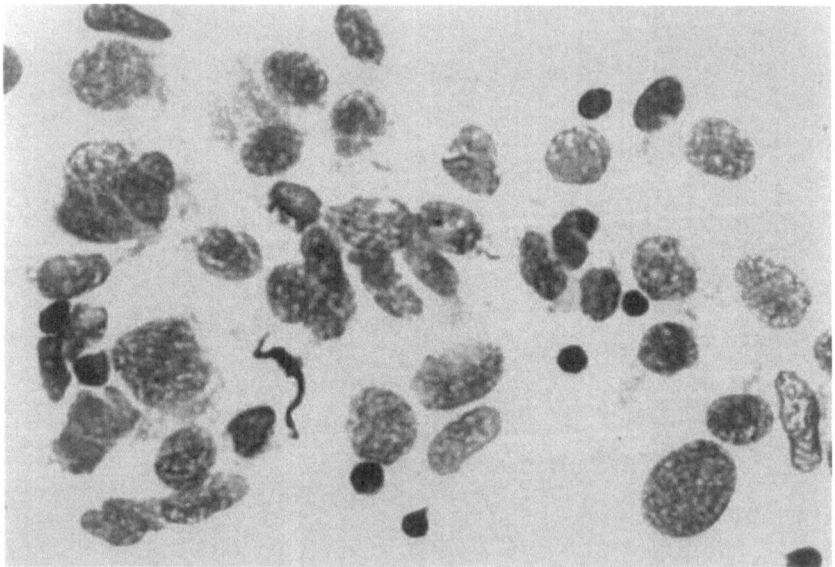

Figure 225 A high power view of the above, showing the nuclei which vary in size but have a similar granular chromatin structure and no nucleoli. The nuclear structure is similar to that seen in the small cigar-shaped cells. May-Grünwald-Giemsa stain (× 800)

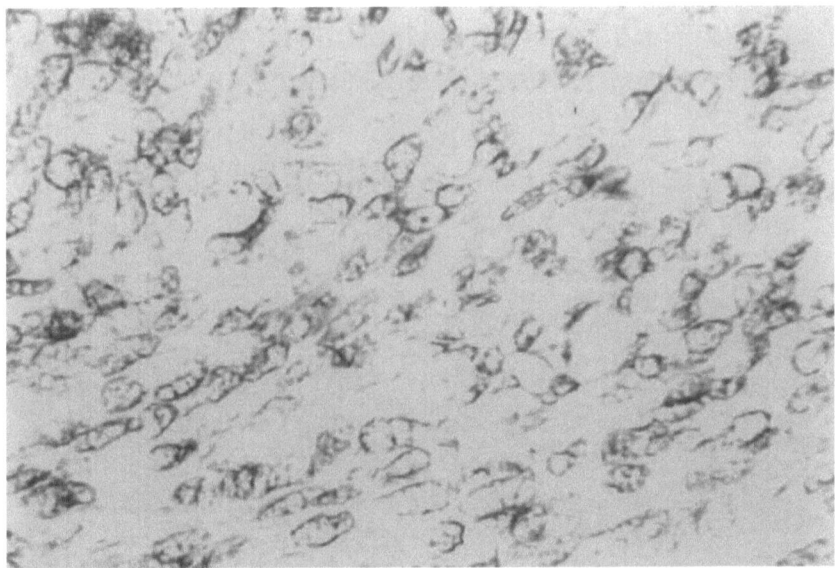

Figure 226 A high power view of a cellular-rich area of connective tissue type cells. May-Grünwald-Giemsa stain (× 730)

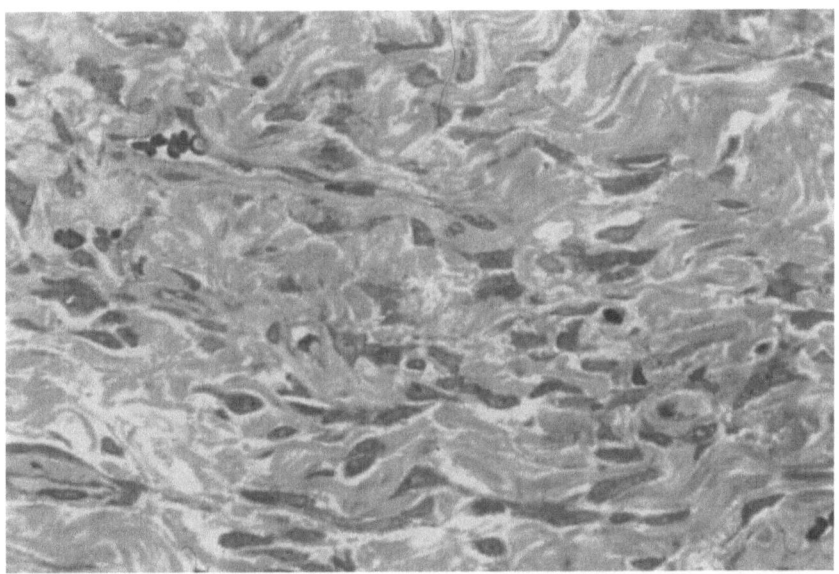

Figure 227 1 µm thick toluidine blue-stained section showing cigar-shaped cells lying within the collagen (× 275)

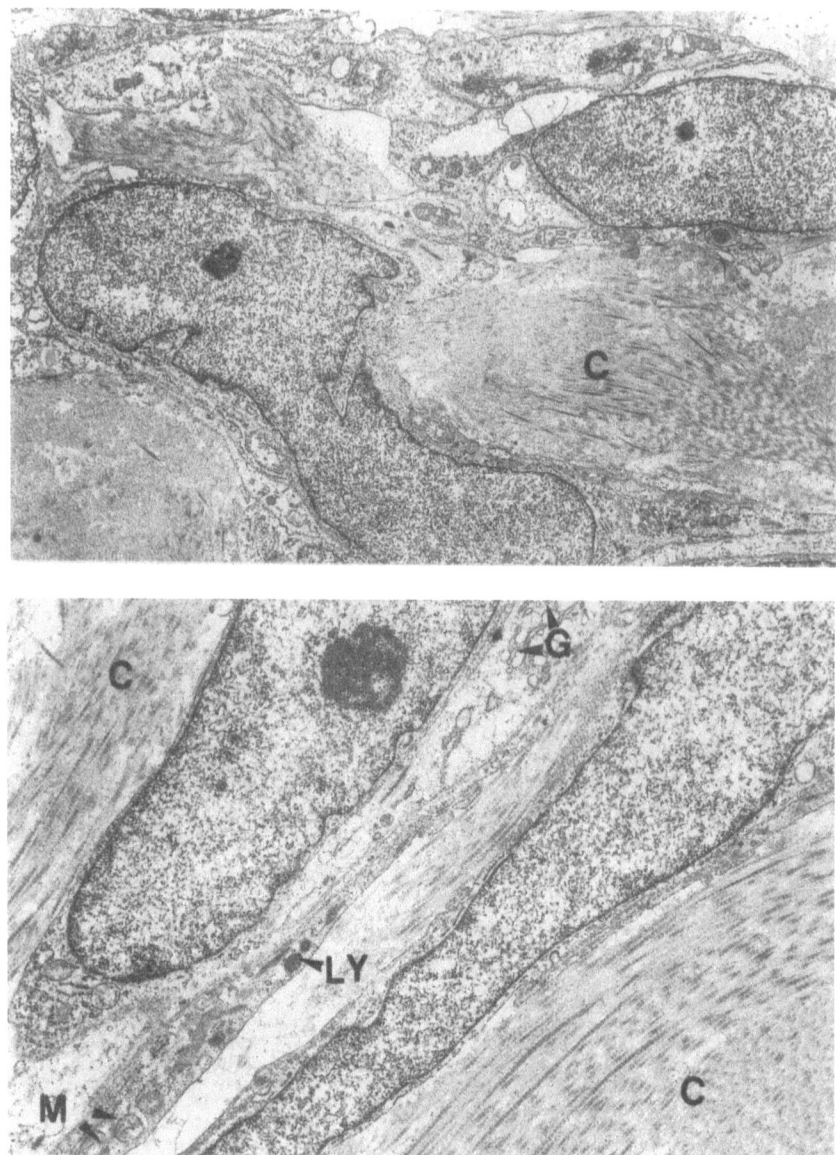

Figures 228 and 229   EM shows the intercellular areas with a granular material composed of typical collagen fibrillae (Figure 228 × 4300, and Figure 229 × 8500)

Key for electron microscope (EM) figures:

C   Collagen
M   Mitochondria
R.E.R.   Rough endoplasmic reticulum
G   Golgi region
Ly   Lysosomes

References

Alvarez-Fernandez, E. and Diez-Nau, M.D. (1979). Malignant fibrosarcomatous mesothelioma and benign fibroma (localized fibrous mesothelioma) in tissue culture. A comparison of the *in vitro* pattern of growth in relation to the cell of origin. *Cancer*, **43**, 1658–1663

Briselli, M., Mark, E.J. and Dickersin, G.R. (1981). Solitary fibrous tumors of the pleura. Eight new cases and review of 360 cases in the literature. *Cancer*, **47**, 2678–2689

Bunton, R.W. and Borrie, D.J. (1982). Pleural fibromas: a clinical review and report of six patients. *Ann.Thorac.Surg.*, **33**, (6), 609–613

Bürrig, K.F., Kastendieck, H. and Hüsselmann, H. (1983). Lokalisierter fibröser Pleuratumor (benignes Mesotheliom). Klinisch-pathologische Untersuchungen an 24 Fällen zur Klassifikation, Morphogenese und Prognose. *Pathologe*, **4**, 120–129

Bürrig, K.-F. and Kastendieck, H. (1984). Ultrastructure observations on the histogenesis of localised fibrous tumours of the pleura (benign mesothelioma). *Virch.Arch.(Pathol.Anat.)*, **403**, 413–424

Enzinger, F.M. and Weiss, S.W. (1983). *Soft Tissue Tumors*, pp. 567–571. (St Louis: C.V. Mosby)

Said, J.W., Nash, G., Banks-Schlegel, S., Sassoon, A.F. and Shintaku, I.P. (1984). Localised fibrous mesothelioma: an immunohistochemical and electron microscopic study. *Hum. Pathol.*, **15**, 440–443

Scharifker, D. and Kaneko, M., (1979). Localized fibrous 'mesothelioma' of pleura (submesothelial fibroma). A clinicopathologic study of 18 cases. *Cancer*, **43**, 627–635

Spencer, H. (1977). *Pathology of the Lung*. 3rd Edn. pp. 920–3. (Oxford: Pergamon)

II. BENIGN ADENOMATOID MESOTHELIOMA

Benign adenomatoid mesothelioma of peritoneum and its derivates:

Includes:	Mesothelioma of uterus, adenomatoid tumour of the uterus. Adenomatoid tumour of the epididymis. Extragenital adenomatoid tumour (adrenal, omentum, mesentery). Benign papillary mesothelioma of peritoneum.
Age range:	18–84 years.
Symptoms and signs:	These depend on the localization of the tumour. They may be absent and the tumour may present as an incidental finding.
Gross pathology:	In the uterus these tumours generally look like sub-serosal leiomyomas but they are less demarcated. In the epididymis the lesions are usually small and cystic. In the peritoneal cavity they may appear as multiple papillary growths or cysts.
Histopathology:	The tumour consists of tubular structures covered by mesothelial cells. Several variants are described (adenoid, angiomatoid, solid and cystic). These structures are surrounded by fibrous tissue, by myometrium or are found lying on top of the peritoneum.
Histogenesis:	This is controversial but most recent reports have favoured a mesothelial origin, usually based upon studies of the ultrastructure. This is in accordance with the embryology. Though a benign neoplasm seems the most probable, a reactive process can not be excluded in some cases.
Case history:	A 36-year-old female. A hysterectomy was performed because of pain and metror-

rhagia. The uterus weighed 100 g and contained several leiomyomas. There was a nodule 1 cm diameter immediately under the serosal surface. Microscopically the nodule consisted of myometrium in which many adenomatoid structures, covered with mesothelial cells were present.

Acknowledgement: This case was kindly contributed by Dr T.L. Ceelen.

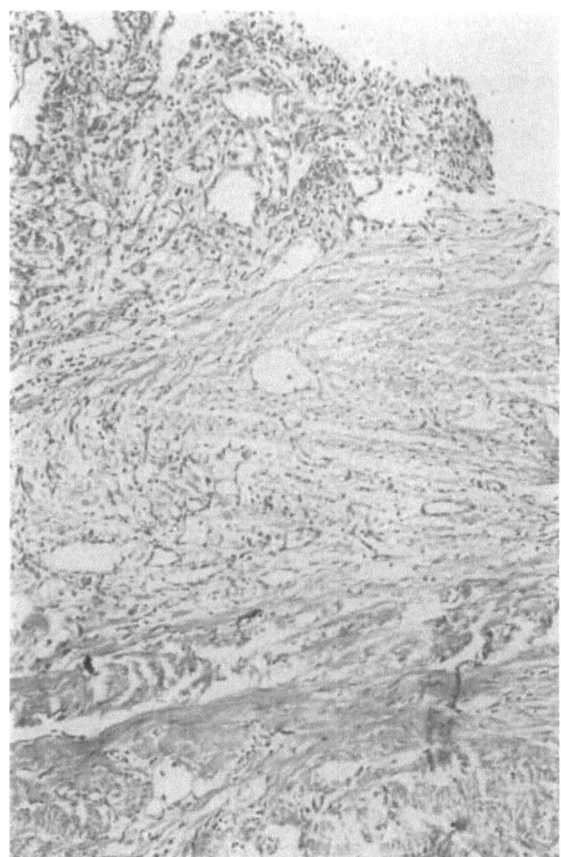

Figure 230 A papillary mesothelial proliferation is arising on the serosal surface of the uterus. Tubules lined by a single layer of cells are present within the subserosal connective tissue (× 110)

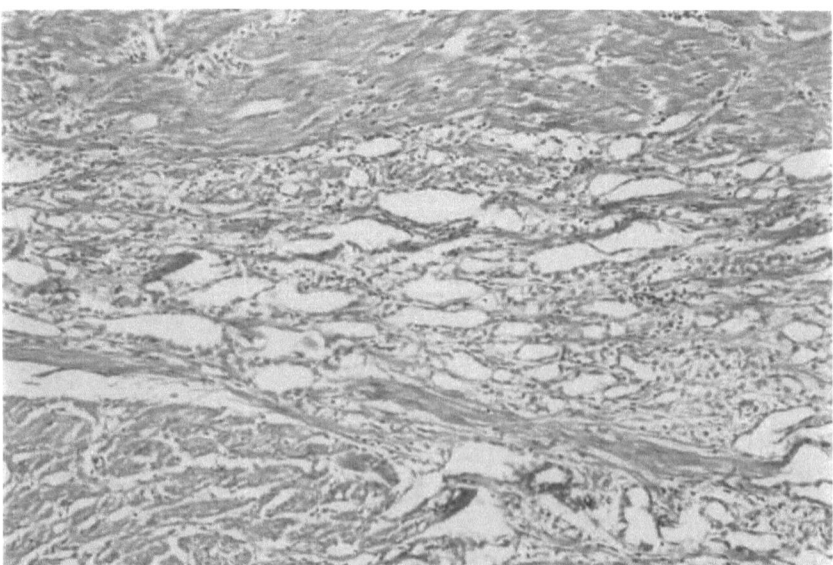

Figure 231 A higher magnification of the nodule in the myometrium shows bundles of smooth muscle with clefts and tubules lined by cuboidal or flattened cells (× 110)

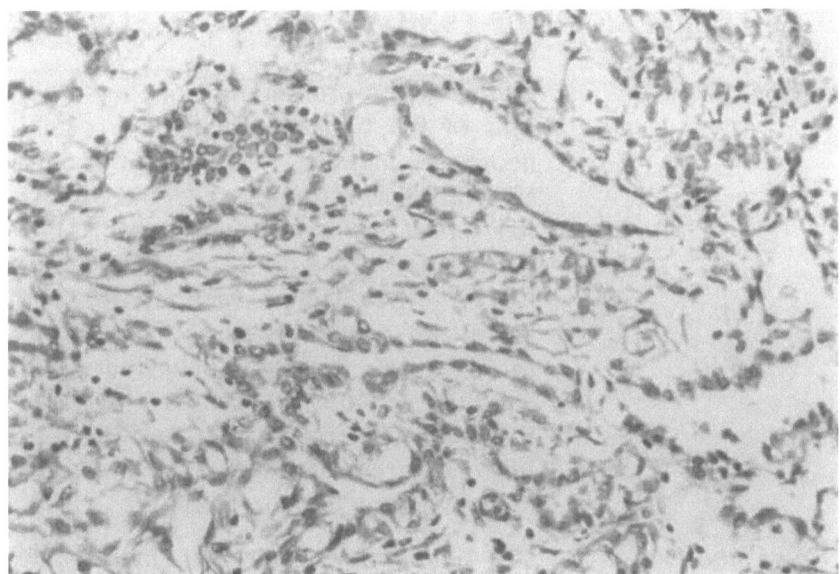

Figure 232 A higher magnification to show the detailed structure of the tubules and clefts (× 275)

References

Addis, B.J. and Fox, H. (1983). Papillary mesothelioma of ovary. *Histopathology,* **7,** 287–298

Craig, J.R. and Hart, W.R. (1979). Extragenital adenomatoid tumor. *Cancer,* **43,** 1678–1681

Davy, C.L. and Tang, C.K. (1981). Are all adenomatoid tumors adenomatoid mesotheliomas? *Hum.Pathol.,* **12,** 360–369

Enzinger, F.M. and Weiss, S.W. (1983). *Soft Tissue Tumors,* pp. 575–576. (St Louis: C.V. Mosby)

Goepel, J.R. (1981) Benign papillary mesothelioma of peritoneum. *Histopathology,* **5,** 21–30

Quigley, J.C. and Hart, W.R. (1981). Adenomatoid tumors of the uterus. *Am.J.Clin.Pathol.,* **76,** 627–635

Said, J.W., Nash, G. and Lee, M. (1982). Immunoperoxidase localization of keratin proteins, carcinoembryonic antigen, and factor VIII in adenomatoid tumors. *Hum.Pathol.,* **13,** 1106–1108

Söderström, K.O. (1982). Origin of adenomatoid tumor. *Cancer,* **49,** 2349–2357

Wood, C. and Bouchelle, W.H. (1978). Benign mesothelioma simulating a uterine leiomyoma. *Am. J.Obstet.Gynaecol.,* **132,** 225–226

III. MESOTHELIOMA OF TUNICA VAGINALIS TESTIS

Natural history:

In rare cases proliferation of the serosal cells of the tunica vaginalis may exhibit neoplastic features. They can be seen in connection with a hydrocoele, but whether this is *post* or *propter* is not known. There is no connection with a testicular tumour. Only a few cases have been reported with asbestos exposure. Because this is such a rare lesion the biological behaviour of this condition cannot be properly assessed. Cases of recurrence after several years have been reported, and some have run a malignant course.

Gross pathology:

The tumour may appear as small papilliferous excrescences of the tunica vaginalis, projecting into the cavity.

Differential diagnosis:

Reactive proliferation of the serosal cells.

Histopathology:

Serosal cells are seen proliferating on a peduncular fibrous stroma forming sessile papillary structures. Invasive growth may be present. The cells are morphologically and also ultrastructurally similar to proliferating mesothelial cells of epithelial type. Under the surface cell layer, characteristic foamy cells are often seen. These cells seem to be variants of mesothelioma cells.

Case history:

A 58-year-old man. He was a farmer with no past history of asbestos exposure. For 5 years he had a left-sided hydrocoele of increasing size. In March 1978 surgical exploration showed a hydrocoele containing 250 ml of serous fluid. The tunica vaginalis was covered by multiple papilliferous excrescences between 2 and 6 mm diameter. No evidence of invasion was seen. No metastatic tumour deposits were identified. An orchidectomy was carried out and the patient made an uneventful recovery.

Acknowledgement: This case was kindly contributed by Dr Svend Aage Askjær.

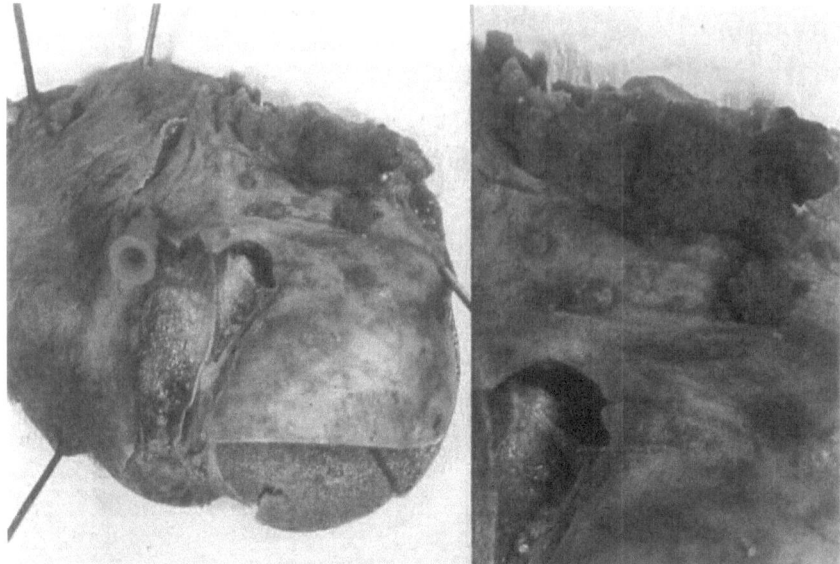

Figure 233 Orchidectomy specimen. On the left is the testis with a distended tunica vaginalis due to a hydrocoele. Several brown papillary excrescences are seen on the surface of the tunica vaginalis. The picture on the right shows a magnified view of the excrescences

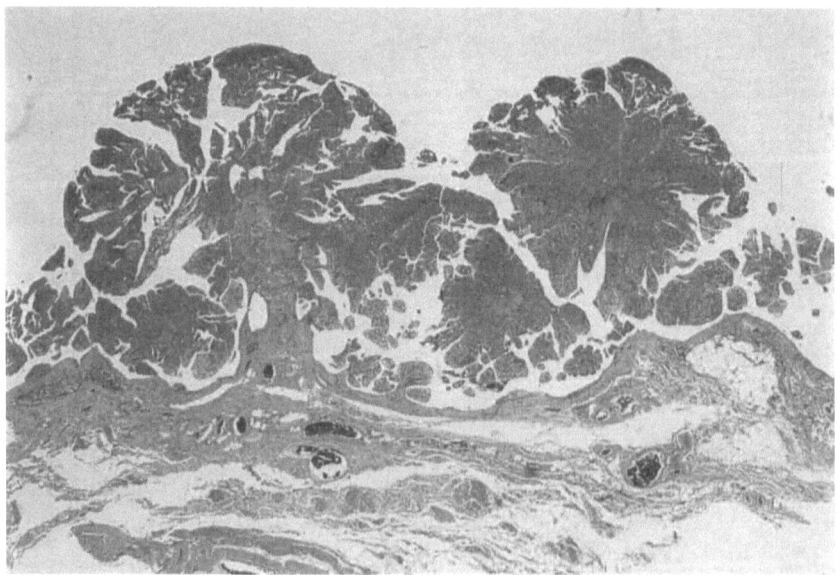

Figure 234 Low power view of a histological section of the papillary excrescenes (× 10)

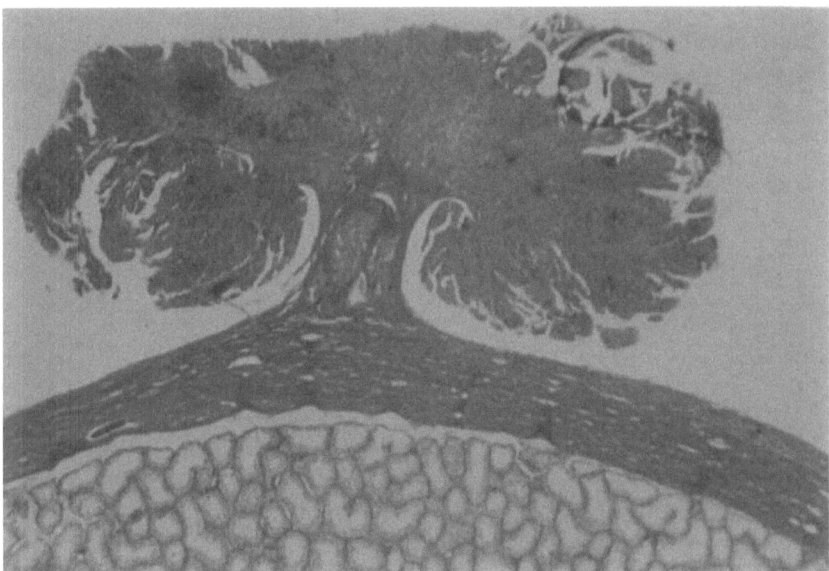

Figure 235 A single papillary tumour arising from the tunica vaginalis. There is no connection through the tunica vaginalis to the underlying testicular tissue. Van Gieson stain (× 16)

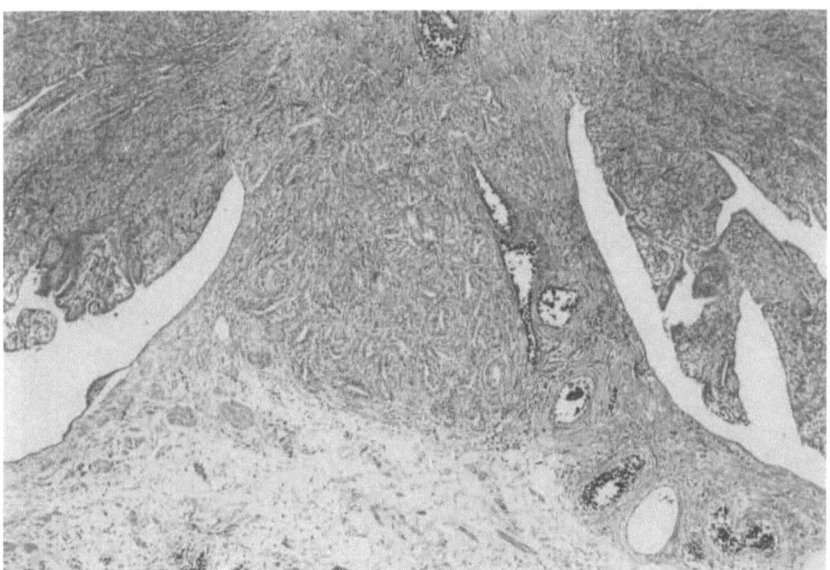

Figure 236 A higher power view of a stalk showing the presence of tumour towards the base (× 45)

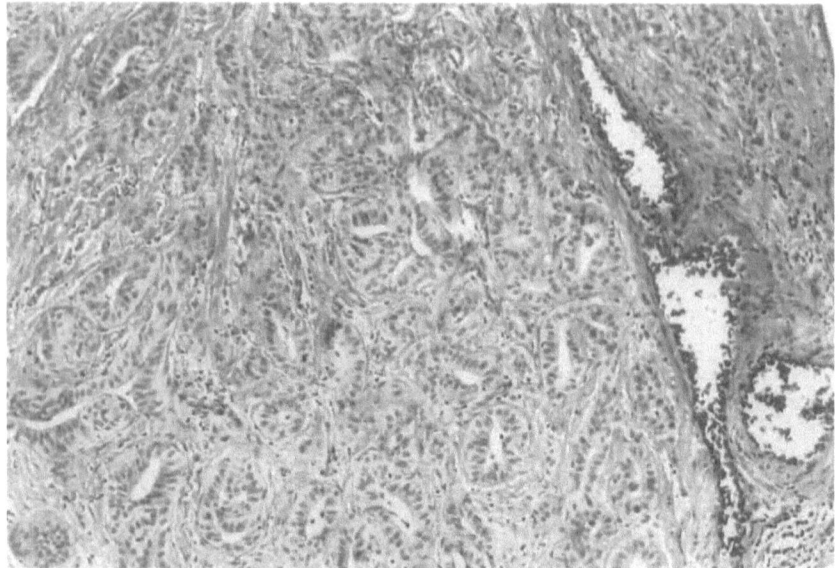

Figure 237 A higher power view of the stalk showing numerous closely packed tubules in a connective tissue stroma (× 110)

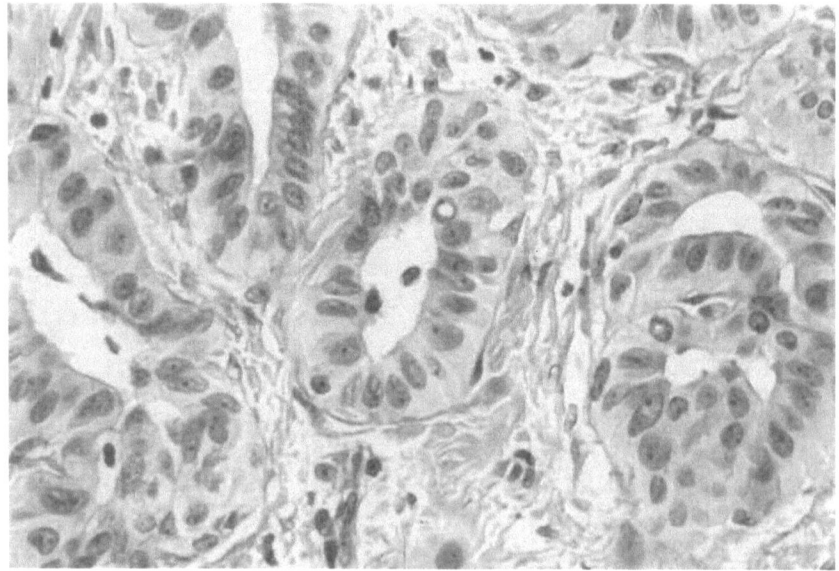

Figure 238 A higher power view of the tubules within the stalk showing the lining of tall columnar cells (× 430)

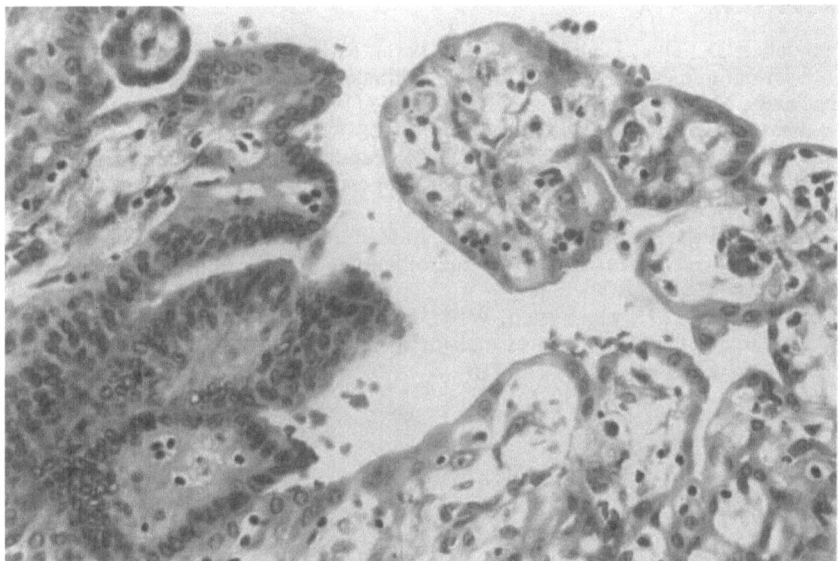

Figure 239   The outer papillary surface of the tumour showing the variation of the covering cells from flattened to tall columnar. Another characteristic feature is the presence of large pale cells with small shrunken nuclei (× 275)

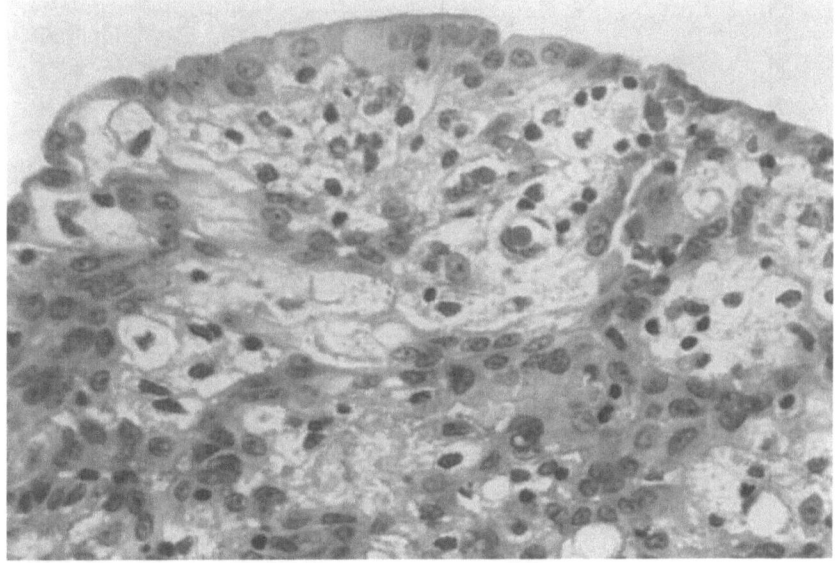

Figure 240   A higher power view of above (× 430)

References

Bandelier, D., Duc, J. and Loosli, H. (1981). Mésothéliome papillaire du cordon spermatique gauche et de la tunique vaginale. *Helv.Chir.Acta,* **48,** 369–375

Hollands, M.J., Dottori, V. and Nach, A.G. (1982). Malignant mesothelioma of the tunica vaginalis testis. *Eur.Urol.,* **8,** 121–122

Mikuz, G. and Höpfel-Kreiner, I. (1982). Papillary mesothelioma of the tunica vaginalis propria testis. Case report and ultrastructural study. *Virch.Arch.Pathol.Anat.,* **396,** 231–238

Japko, L., Horta, A.A., Schreiber, K., Mitsudo, S., Karwa, G.L., Singh, G. and Koss, L.G. (1982). Malignant mesothelioma of the tunica vaginalis testis. *Cancer,* **49,** 119–127

van der Rhee, H.J., van Vloten, W.A., Scheffer, E. and Zwartendyk, J. (1983). Cutaneous manifestations of malignant mesothelioma of the tunica vaginalis testis. *J.Cut.Pathol.,* **10,** 213–216

IV. MESOTHELIOMA OF A–V NODE

Synonyms: Coelothéliome Tawarien benin.
Congenital polycystic tumour of the atrio-ventricular node.
Epithelial heterotopia.
Endodermal inclusions.

Age range and sex: The age range is from newborn to the 9th decade, one half dying before the age of 30. The male/female ratio is 1 to 2.5.

Symptoms and signs: Partial or total heart block and sometimes sudden unexpected death are the main features.

Gross pathology: A cystic tumour of varying size in the region of the A–V node may be found, but small tumours may be invisible to the naked eye.

Histopathology: The A–V node is more or less replaced by tubules and/or cystic spaces, mostly filled with intra- and extra-cellular PAS-positive material, which may be diastase-resistant. The cellular lining may be flattened, cuboidal or cylindrical, and sometimes squamoid. There is a varying amount of loose fibrovascular connective tissue with scattered chronic inflammatory cells. All the histological features are benign.

Histogenesis: This is still under debate. At present an origin either from sequestered endodermal elements or from epicardial mesoderm is favoured, but neither of these theories is conclusively established. The constant presence of diastase PAS-positive material is not in favour of a mesothelial origin and the lesion could be considered a hamartoma rather than a true neoplasm.

Case history: 37-year-old man of unknown occupation. No pre-existing cardiac symptoms. He developed chest pain, and an E.C.G. tracing revealed partial A–V block. Sudden death occurred one week later. Autopsy revealed a macroscopically normal heart (340 g) with only minor atherosclerosis of the coronary arteries. In particular there was no tumour in the region of the A–V node on naked eye examination. Microscopy of the conducting system however revealed evidence of tumour in three out of six blocks from the A–V node region. The rest of the conducting system was normal.

Acknowledgement: This case was kindly contributed by Dr Jens Vilhelm Thorborg.

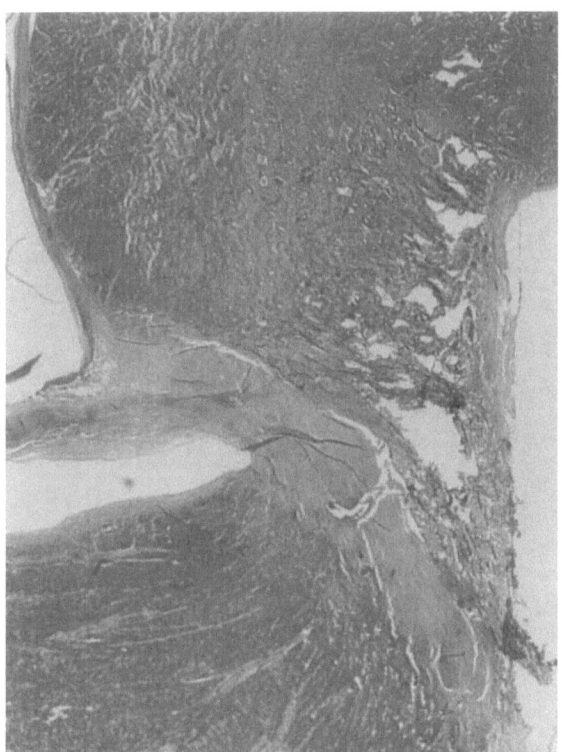

Figure 241 A low power view of the A–V groove with the atrium above and the ventricle below. In the lower part of the atrial wall the tumour is seen as an area of faint pallor on the right side (× 8)

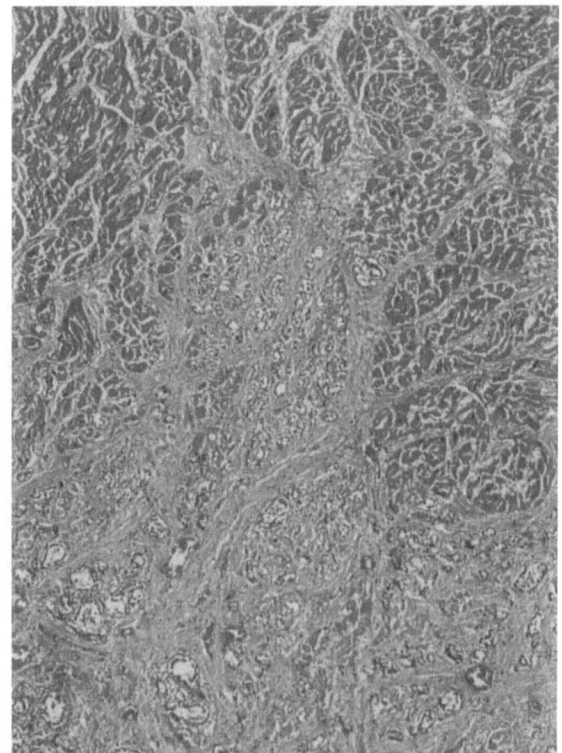

Figure 242 A more detailed view of the tumour to show it dividing bundles of myocardium (× 45)

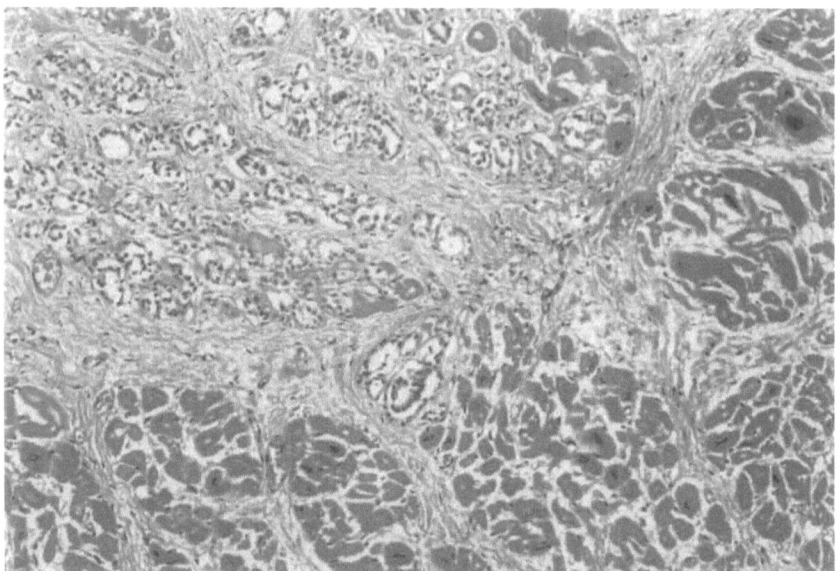

Figure 243 A higher power view showing the tumour to be composed of tubules and small cysts in a cellular-poor fibrotic stroma (× 110)

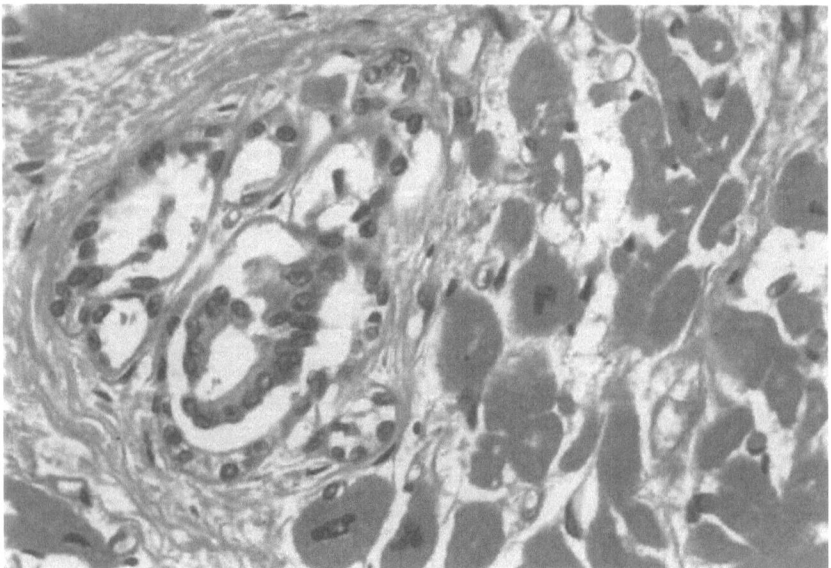

Figure 244 A higher power view of above showing the tubules to be lying within the myocardium. The fibrous stroma and atrophic myocardial fibres are seen in the vicinity of the tubules (× 430)

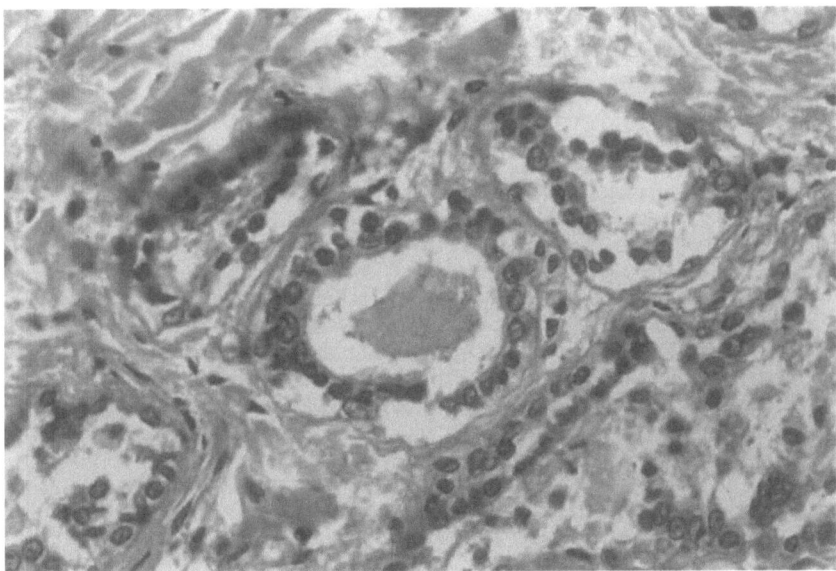

Figure 245   The tubules are lined by low columnar cells and the lumen contains uniformly staining eosinophilic material (× 430)

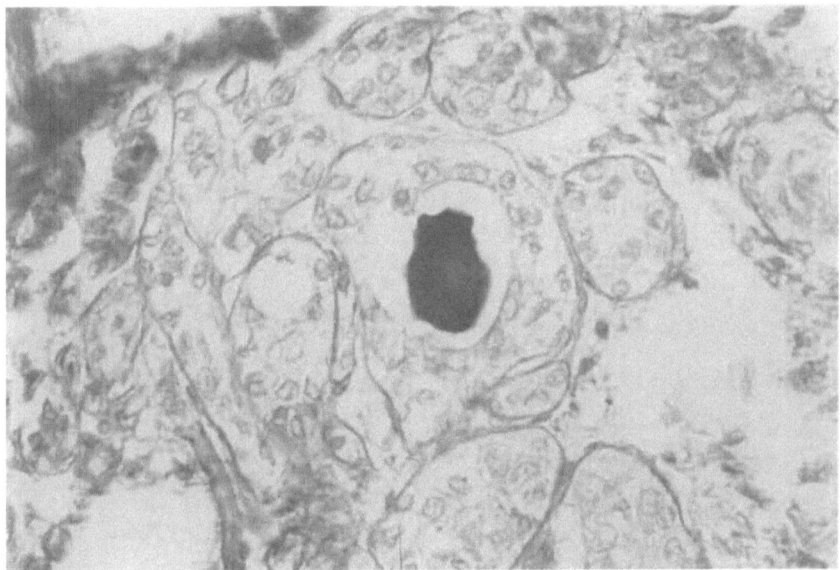

Figure 246   Diastase–PAS staining shows this material to be strongly positive (× 430)

References

Castleman, B., Scully, R.E. and McNeely, B.U. (1973). Case records of the Massachusetts General Hospital, Case 6. *N.Engl.J.Med.*, **288**, 308–315

Castleman, B., Scully, R.E. and McNeely, B.U. (1982). Case records of the Massachusetts General Hospital, *N.Engl.J.Med.*, **306**, 32–39

Lie, J.T., Lufrikanowski, R. and Erickson, E.E. (1980). Heterotopic epithelial replacement (so-called 'mesothelioma') of the atrioventricular node, congenital heart block and sudden death. *Am.J.Forensic Med.Pathol.*, **1/2**, 131–137

Mahaim, I. (1945). *Les Tumeurs et les Polypes du Coeur*. pp 246–77. (Paris: Masson and Cie)

Paulsen, S.M. and Kristensen, I.B. (1981). So-called mesothelioma of the atrioventricular node. *J. Submicrosc. Cytol.*, **13**, 667–674

Travers, H. (1982). Congenital polycystic tumor of the atrioventricular node; possible familial occurrence and critical review of reported cases with special emphasis on histogenesis. *Hum. Pathol.*, **13**, 25–35

Bibliography

Asbestos Associated Diseases, Special Issue. *Arch. Pathol. Lab. Med.,* Vol. 106, (11), October 1982

Asbestos edited by L. Michaels and S.S. Chissick (1979). (Chichester, New York, Brisbane, Toronto: John Wiley)

Asbestos and Disease by I.J. Selikoff and D.H. Lee (1978). (New York, San Fransisco, London: Academic Press)

Asbestos and Mesothelioma, A Review, M. Kannerstein, J. Churg, and W.T.E. McCaughey (1978), *Pathol. Ann.,* **13,** 81–129

Asbest und Mesotheliom by H. Bohlig and H. Otto (1975). (Stuttgart: Georg Thieme Verlag)

Asbestos, Vol. 1 and 2. Final report of the advisory committee, Health and Safety Commission (1979). (London: Her Majesty's Stationery Office)

Biological Effects of Asbestos edited by P. Bogovski, J.C. Gilson, V. Timbrell and J.C. Wagner (1973). I.A.R.C. Scientific Publications No. 8, Lyon

Biological Effects of Mineral Fibres edited by J.C. Wagner (1980). I.A.R.C. Scientific Publications No. 30. INSERM Symposia Series Volume 92, Lyon

Current Concepts, Malignant Mesothelioma, K.H. Antman (1980). *N. Engl. J. Med.,* **303,** 200–202

Health Hazards of Asbestos Exposure edited by Selikoff, I.J. and Hammond, E.C. (1979). *Ann. N.Y. Acad. Sci. 330*

Malignant Mesothelioma 1982: Review of 4710 published cases. G. Hillerdal (1983). *Br.J.Dis.Chest,* **77,** 321–343

Pathology Annual 1982. Part 2, Vol. 17. Current Problems in Pathology of Asbestos-related Disease. A. Churg and J. Golden

Seminars in Oncology, Asbestos-related Neoplasms edited by J.W. Yarbro, J. Aisner and P.H. Wiernik (1981). **VIII,** No. 3

Soft Tissue Tumors F.M. Enzinger and S.W. Weiss (1983). (St Louis: C.V. Mosby)

Index

In this index the term *mesothelioma* indicates *diffuse malignant mesothelioma*. Other forms are referred to in full, eg. *localized mesothelioma, benign*.